# Kripalu's
# *Self Health*
# *Guide*

**A Personal Program
for Holistic Living**

**Illustrators, Designers, and Editors, First Edition:**
Carolyn Delluomo
Lesley Dove
Carol Finnegan
David Jackson
Laura Moore
William Nuessle, Ph.D.
Don Stapleton, Ph.D.
Jane Yelland

**Illustrators, Designers, and Editors, Revised Edition:**
Linda Cutler
Toni Kenny
Kent Lew
Lorraine Nelson
Dennis Slattery
Michael Vuksta

**Photographs, Revised Edition:**
Adam Mastoon
Sheila Richards
Patricia Seip
Ron King

**Special Note:**
Most photographs are of the grounds of Kripalu Center for Yoga and Health or of program participants or residents at the Center.

Kripalu Publications
P.O. Box 793, Lenox, MA 01240

© 1980, 1993
by Kripalu Yoga Fellowship

Published 1980
Second Printing 1981
Third Printing 1984
Revised Edition 1993

"Kripalu" is a registered trademark of Kripalu Yoga Fellowship.

Library of Congress
Catalog Card Number: 93-78262
ISBN 0-940258-28-5

# Kripalu's *Self Health Guide*

## A Personal Program for Holistic Living

## Revised Edition

Compiled by the staff of
Kripalu Center for Yoga and Health,
based on the teachings of Yogi Amrit Desai

Kripalu Publications
Lenox, MA

# Table of Contents

# The Fourth Pathway: learning the art of relaxed work

# The Fifth Pathway: discovering your optimum diet

# The Sixth Pathway: mastering communication — with yourself and others

# The Seventh Pathway: practicing meditation and spiritual attunement

# The Eighth Pathway: creating a supportive lifestyle

# Appendix

Your own body is the very best book on health
that you will ever read.

# *Introduction*
## about this book

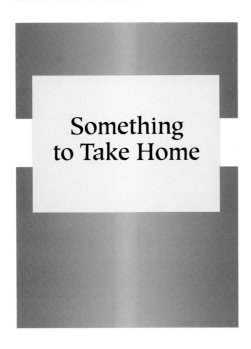

## Something to Take Home

Soon after Kripalu Center for Yoga and Health opened, guests who came for programs were asking for something to take home to continue the personal growth work they had begun here.

Many lived far away and could come to the Center only occasionally. Others wanted to share what they had learned here with relatives and friends who had never heard of Kripalu. All were looking for ways to make the Kripalu Approach to health a part of their daily lives.

Our response to their requests is *Kripalu's Self Health Guide: A Personal Program for Holistic Living.* Based on materials used in our programs, it is filled not only with information and inspiration, but with self-discovery experiences and introspections that can help change your life, just as the lives of visitors to Kripalu Center have been changed.

It is our hope that your use of the exercises we have provided in *Kripalu's Self Health Guide* will lead you to insights and experiences of yourself that are so deep that they bring about a permanent trans-for-mation of the way you experience your life.

The first chapter of *Kripalu's Self Health Guide* gives an overview of ways of looking at health and wholeness and introduces the Kripalu Approach to holistic health. The basic premise of the Kripalu Approach is that we each have an inner wisdom that will take us to wholeness if we can learn how to listen to and follow it. The chapter also includes a Holistic Health Appraisal Checklist that helps you to see where you are now in your habits and attitudes about health.

Once you begin to have a picture of what high-level well-being could look like for you and an idea of where you are right now, the next question is "How do I get there from here?"

In the second chapter we offer our answer to that question: the Kripalu Approach. It is a practical program utilizing natural tools and techniques of healing from East and West that can work for everyone to bring about a more harmonious lifestyle and greater levels of health and wholeness. The Kripalu Approach is organized into eight pathways, which correspond to the eight major ways in which we express our energy in daily living and interact with the energy within us. In the remainder of the book, each pathway is explored at length, using three kinds of material designed to make your learning enjoyable and experiential.

Essays describing the basic principles and theory of the Kripalu Approach are the first kind of material. Many of the essays are by Yogi Amrit Desai, the founder and spiritual director of Kripalu Center. The remainder are from materials used in programs at Kripalu.. They reflect Yogi Desai's teachings as well as other ancient and modern, Eastern and Western sources.

Secondly, there are what we call Self-Discovery Experiences that help you discover where you are now in relation to the principles of the Kripalu Approach and to your desired health goals. Finally, there are "How To" sections containing practical ideas, exercises, and techniques designed to help you put into practice all that you learn.

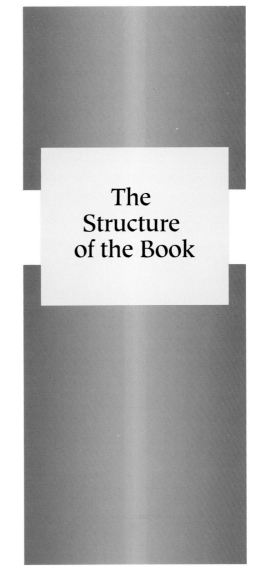

## The Structure of the Book

Reading a book does not as a rule put us in touch with our experience; more often than not it takes us out of the sensations we are experiencing and into thinking about them. In the area of personal growth and development, experience is the best teacher.

According to developmental psychologists, we learn more in the first few years of our lives than in all the remaining years, because at that early age we learn experientially rather than intellectually. That is the first reason we have included self-discovery experiences.

The second reason is that the Kripalu Approach as we teach it in our programs is based on experiential learning. As a visitor to Kripalu Center, you would find that a central ingredient in all our programs is guided experience. This book has been designed to bring you an approximation of some of the experiences you might have if you came here.

The third reason is that personal experiences are just more fun! It is much more interesting and real to experience something for yourself than simply to have it explained to you.

# Kripalu "Self-Discovery Experiences"

And why do we call them "self" discovery experiences? Because many of us do not always know what feelings we are experiencing as we confront certain issues in our lives. We believe that what we think is what we feel. Even when we do get in touch with our feelings, we are accustomed not to acknowledge them for social or other reasons. So most of us need practice in getting in touch with and expressing our feelings.

The introspections, then, are experiences that help you rediscover yourself: what you really think and feel about life and health and yourself. When you know where you stand, you can set off in a direction of your choice, making the changes that feel right to you.

One thing to remember when you do the introspections: it is very important to sit quietly with your eyes closed and become really relaxed before beginning them. Take all the time you need to do that, because it is the relaxed state that allows insights to come to you from a level beyond your conscious, habitual thinking. As you become more adept at the technique, you will be amazed at what you are able to learn from yourself!

This book is intended as a workbook (and a fun book) for you to record your experiences and discoveries. You may prefer not to write in the book itself, and in places you'll probably need more space (especially where we invite you to draw). We recommend that you work in a special notebook or journal, so that the material remains in sequence and does not get separated or scattered as it may if it is on loose sheets. Then you will be able to refer to your notes easily as you monitor your progress.

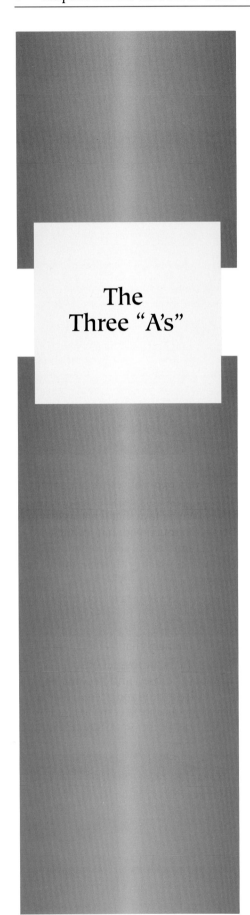

# The Three "A's"

A key part of our approach to self-discovery is what we call "The Three 'A's'": Awareness, Acceptance, and Adjustment. They are the three stages into which the Kripalu Approach divides the process of making desired changes in our lives.

1. *Awareness.* We must know where we are before we can decide how to get where we want to go. Think of setting off in your car to see friends, getting lost, and phoning them for directions. Before they can tell you how to get to their house, the first question they must ask is: "Where are you now?" Once you have a goal, the answer to "Where are you now?" always determines your next move.

2. *Acceptance.* Awareness and acceptance are intertwined. By learning to accept freely and uncritically where we are at this moment, we begin to allow our unconscious to release more and more knowledge about ourselves. The process of acceptance is one of acknowledging to ourselves that where we are is in fact perfect — it is where we are supposed to be right now.

   Mentally fighting our current situation with judgements such as "I should be better" drains our energy and self-esteem. Without acceptance of where we are, there is no possibility of moving in a direction of our choice or of ever enjoying ourselves fully.

   For example, until someone acknowledges and accepts a current situation of being overweight, he or she cannot choose the goal of thinness and enjoy the process of moving toward it.

3. *Adjustment.* Once the two preceding stages have been fully experienced and accepted, we can go on to make the changes in our habits that we desire to make and that will bring us to a state of greater holistic health.

The keys to the stage of Adjustment are patience and moderation. Often, we either go too fast and become discouraged when we can't change everything overnight, or else we think that the changes needed are so great that we'll never be able to make them and discourage ourselves before we start.

The Kripalu Approach recommends gentle, gradual changes, starting with something that we know we will find easy and even pleasant to accomplish. Then, encouraged by our success, we'll feel inspired to continue into slightly more difficult areas. The whole process is a game we play with the subconscious mind, tricking it into giving up its grip on old, non-productive habit patterns.

The three stages of Awareness, Acceptance, and Adjustment are used in each of the eight pathways to health in the Kripalu Approach. They can also be helpful in facilitating any of life's transitions, from changing jobs to dealing with accidents or severe illness. Try them and see how they work for you.

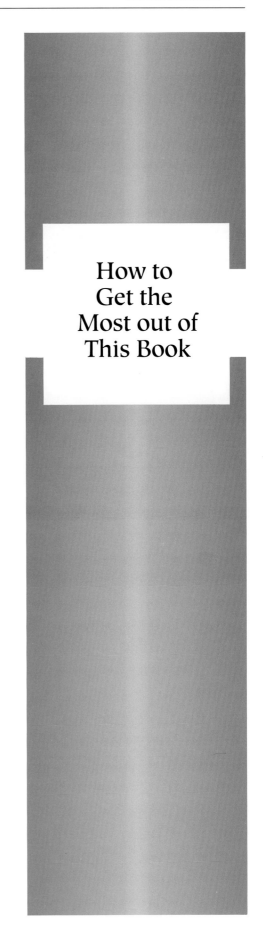

## How to Get the Most out of This Book

1. Use this book, not just to add to your store of intellectual knowledge, but to experience yourself in new ways. Use it as you would a cookbook, where you wouldn't just read the recipes — you'd cook them and enjoy the meals. The meal you will enjoy from totally immersing yourself in this book is a new and exciting experience of yourself that can make your life healthier and happier.

2. Digest the book slowly, chapter by chapter. Continuing the recipe analogy, read as if you are savoring a delicious meal and want to get the most out of every mouthful. Consciously chew well each Self-Discovery portion before going on to the next section of straight reading.

3. Follow the recipes closely. Find a quiet, peaceful, pleasant place to read the book and to do the exercises, so that you can really take in the material and allow it to affect you on a deep level.

4. Observe the way you use this book as another part of the learning it can convey to you. Do you have a tendency to want just to continue reading passively, investing little energy into self-revelation? Or are you eager to complete the Self-Discovery Experiences, actively investing energy to reveal you to yourself? Know that it's fine either way; it simply shows your mood of the moment, so just observe it as more data you're collecting on that most fascinating person: you!

5. Take one step at a time. Select an area where you know you will enjoy working and changing and make a commitment to it. Not only will your success in that area make it easier to commit to working on another, but you will find that your attention to one area causes other changes to occur automatically.

6. Most important, have a good time! More than anything else we want this book to be enjoyable and fun, and a pleasure to read and work with. At Kripalu we have found that getting to know ourselves better is one of the most exhilarating and gratifying experiences of life.

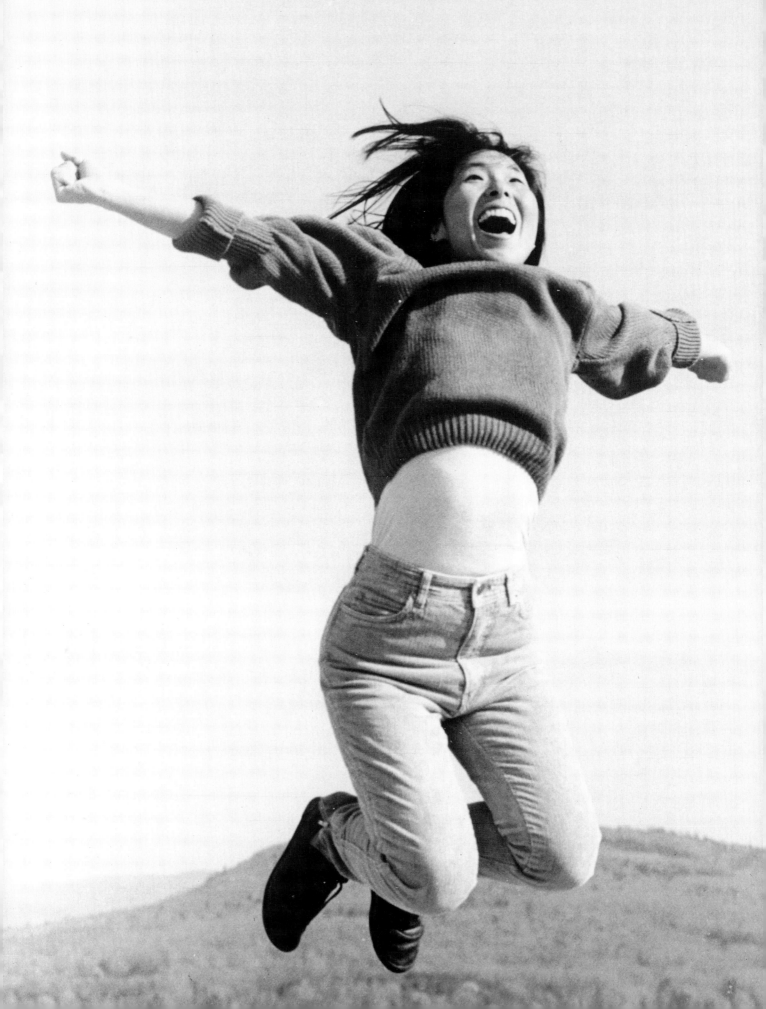

# *The Goal and the Guide*

## a look at health and wholeness

# Holistic Health

Did you know that in the next sixty seconds your heart, an organ about the size of your fist, will pump at least five quarts of blood through sixty thousand miles of veins, arteries, and capillaries? Or that in the space of that same minute, in the routine maintenance of your body, one hundred twenty million new cells will be created, without your having to give them a moment's thought?

Since you are reading this book, you probably realize that an awareness of the miraculous functioning of the human body and its interconnectedness with mind and spirit can greatly improve the quality of your life and health. So, whether or not you use the term "holistic health," you have no doubt embraced in your life many facets of its approach, which affirms that there is more to health than mere absence or avoidance of disease: true health is a state of radiant well-being.

Life, to the holistic health practitioner, is more than just living: it is a celebration of being alive. It is being captivated by nature's supreme craftsmanship evidenced in the human body, mind, and spirit. It is realizing that the body, like the violin of a virtuoso musician, is a delicate and subtle instrument that must be handled with the greatest care and respect and tuned with deep sensitivity before the music of life can pour from it with beauty and harmony.

Holistic health invites us to activate our ability to be the artist and creator of our own life and health. It invites us to recognize that, by first creating harmony within our own body, mind, and spirit, we become co-creators in the great symphony of life rather than merely humming a pleasant but out-of-tune melody. Holistic health invites us to affirm nature's miraculous artistry in us by attaining the high level of radiant health, inner peace, and joyful spiritual well-being for which we were born.

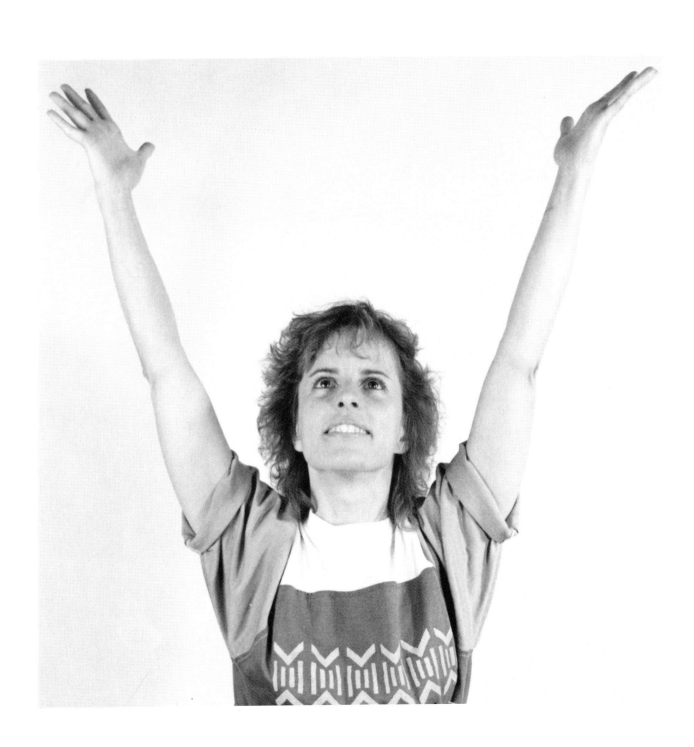

## What Does It Mean to Be Healthy?

Most of us have grown up with a perception of health that is limited by the current dictionary definition as "the condition of being sound in body, mind, or soul; especially freedom from physical disease or pain" (Webster). However, if you look at the roots of the word, you see that originally it included a great deal more.

The word *health* comes from the Old English word *hal*, which means "whole." *Holy*, the condition "characterized by perfection and transcendence" (Webster) also comes from that root. And, together with the word *holistic* or *holism*, they have a common ancestry in the primal Greek root *holos*, which again means "whole."

Those root meanings suggest that to our ancestors health meant being whole. So we shortchange ourselves if we think of health merely as the physical state of not feeling ill. The approach of holistic health seeks to provide what the Greeks had in mind: the experience of wholeness that borders on "hol-i-ness," with the trinity of body, mind, and spirit vibrating to its full health potential.

Yogi Amrit Desai has summed up the holistic approach as follows: "Awakening the body to its higher potentials, in cooperation with a healthy mind, is the beginning of holistic health. Then the higher consciousness naturally emerges within you." Such a definition of health is much beyond the scope of a successful physical exam and could hardly be measured by it!

The question is, are we willing to broaden our image of health and affirm that "Yes, health is more than the absence of disease; it is more than eating right, quitting smoking, or running every day. True health involves all that I think, feel, say, and do. It is the harmonious interaction of all parts of me: my body, mind, and spirit. It is the experience of wholeness and therefore not just the maintenance but the celebration of my self, my universe, and my life."

## Settling for Second Best

When you examine your definition of health and the degree to which your actions are consistent with that definition, you may find that you have settled for second best. Even if you believe true health to be the experience of vibrant well-being, you may still be defining well-being as simply the absence of disease.

When we believe, as most of us have been taught, that we "catch" a cold and should "cure" our ailments by taking medication, we are unconsciously subscribing to a definition of health that merely maintains life, rather than celebrating it.

Those perceptions and actions have their roots in what has been the conventional model of health care since the time of Louis Pasteur in the mid-1800's. His microbiological interpretation demonstrated the existence of germs and their relation to disease.

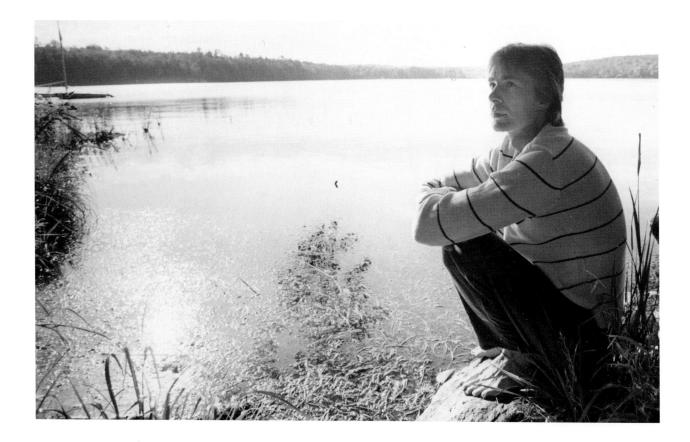

The germ theory, as it was called, quickly found its way into our medical systems until the health field became dominated by the belief that if germs could be controlled or destroyed, the consequent experience was one of health. The result was again a second-best definition of health: "I am well if my doctor says I'm not ill."

## Hygea and Panacea

In ancient Greece there were two schools of thought in regard to health that philosophically reflect our conventional and holistic models. The goddess Panacea ruled over the domain of healing and represented the approach of making a wrong (an illness) right, while Hygea was the goddess of health through appropriate living. The holistic approach suggests a return to the domain of Hygea, of enjoying health by involving all our energy — physical, mental, and spiritual — in attuning our lives to nature's laws.

Take a look now at the chart below which compares the holistic and conventional models. Notice the actions and perceptions that most closely approximate your own steps toward health. Notice the claim of holism that it is not merely a germ that is responsible for our lack of health and it is not our physician who is responsible for making us healthy. It is we, ourselves, who are ultimately responsible for the level at which we are in harmony with the health-sustaining laws of nature.

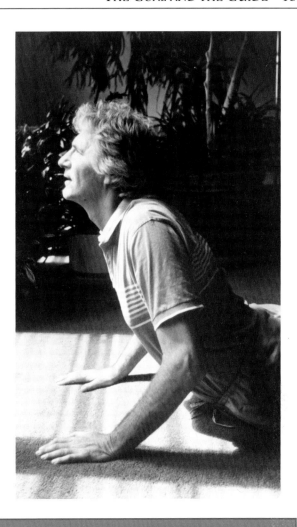

## A Comparison of the Conventional and Holistic Health Care Models

### Conventional Health Care

Looks at diseases and symptoms

Cares for body and mind

Aims at normal health, i.e., absence of disease

Treats symptoms of body and mind by separate specialists

Focuses on treatment and cure

Is for crisis intervention

Is based mainly on drug or surgical intervention

Is based on theory and scientific proof

Sees patient as passive, unknowledgeable recipient of cure

Is based on conventional allopathic methods

### Holistic Health Care

Looks at whole person

Cares for body, mind, and spirit

Aims at high-level vibrant energy

Integrates treatment of body, mind, and spirit

Focuses on prevention and education

Is for ongoing maintenance of health

Is based on natural methods of restoring balance wherever possible

Accepts experiential and intuitive approaches

Recognizes individual's right and ability to take responsibility for own healing process

Utilizes non-conventional and homeopathic methods where appropriate

# The Kripalu Approach to Health

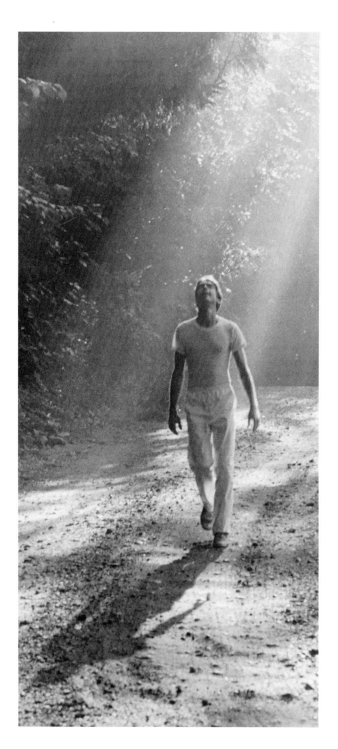

The Kripalu Approach to health is based on two fundamental principles. The first is expressed in the opening quotation of this book: "Your own body is the best book on health you will ever read." Those words were spoken by Yogi Amrit Desai, who went on to ask: "But do you know how to read it?"

In the Kripalu Approach we learn how to focus attention on the experience of our bodies, using our interpretation of that experience as our own personalized path to vibrant health and well-being. We thus begin by turning inward, observing ourselves and the ways we experience our lives.

Next we are asked to make a strong affirmation: "I accept my present state of health and well-being with its weak spots. I recognize that I have created my health, consciously or unconsciously, and I take responsibility for it. I create my life's experiences and where I am right now is exactly where I need to be to learn about life and health."

We know the ground on which we are standing and integrate the wisdom that comes from the lessons of our experience thus far.

The second basic principle of the Kripalu Approach is that we in this three-dimensional, seemingly solid form are expressions of the energy of life and that everything we say and do is an expression of our own inner life energy — of spending or conserving it.

Our present state of well-being is a result of how we have used that energy in the past. It is not a question of judging as good or bad the ways in which we have used our energy; we acted with the awareness that was available to us at the time. Now we can make different choices if we wish as we begin to see how our lives work in terms of energy. To see that, we need to understand what the Kripalu Approach calls "the principle of prana."

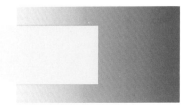

# The Principle of Prana

The wisdom on which our life depends has never come to us through verbal information; it is the wisdom of *prana*, the life force within us that activates all the functions of the body. Guided by its own innate intelligence, prana flows through the nerve currents of the body as a conscious energy and carries out millions of intricate life-giving processes with precise order and intelligence.

Prana's wisdom is known by many names: body instinct, wisdom of the body, inner voice, involuntary nervous system, intuition, and inner guidance. Whatever name we choose, the wisdom of prana is far superior to any other knowledge that we have today. Even in this age of advanced science and technology, we have failed to comprehend fully or reproduce what prana accomplishes daily within our bodies.

We never had to learn how to breathe, circulate our blood, digest our food, eliminate poisons, or heal our bodies, because the life force of prana with its unparalleled and often incomprehensible intelligence carries out all such complex processes for us from birth to death. Ignoring this inner wisdom is the root cause of all disease; listening to its unerring advice is the best program of holistic health available to us.

Yogi Amrit Desai describes prana as the inner energy, the individual manifestation of the life force, that accomplishes our essential life functions without our having to direct it consciously. Prana can also help us accomplish, in a way that is attuned to the greater life energy, functions that are not automatic, but require conscious decisions — when and how much to eat or sleep, for example.

Prana speaks to us through our intuition, our inner sense of knowing what is right or wrong for our bodies at any given time. But prana can be ignored, and many of us have ignored it for so long that it has become a lost language we have forgotten how to read.

Most of us have experienced moments when we sat down to a meal and ate, not because we were hungry, but because it was delicious. In doing that, we ignored prana. Or perhaps one night we were very sleepy, but a friend called and we went to a movie anyway. Our tiredness was prana's way of speaking to us, saying we needed sleep. Again, we ignored it.

If we do not listen to prana, we miss the opportunity of experiencing the balance and inner harmony that is our birthright. We do a disservice to ourselves as whole beings, not just to our bodies. If we ignore prana habitually and often enough, we create the state of dis-ease in the body, a disharmony between body, mind, and emotions and prana.

When our prana is depleted, we become restless and negative in our outlook on life. Our imagination becomes limited; our creativity is impaired; we cannot think clearly. We have no zest, no energy, no vitality. Faced with that condition, prana will seek to fulfill its natural role of homeostasis, of restoring us to ease, but only our listening and responding will make healing possible.

The source of our health is nowhere else but within us. We can read all sorts of books on health, but they won't help until we know how to read our own bodies and the signals of prana. Then illness becomes a messenger of prana, a telegram saying that somewhere in our lives we have lost balance. And prana is a diagnostic center within us, our own holistic health handbook, to which we can go for guidance.

So the purpose of the Kripalu Approach to health is beyond having a finely-tuned body and a calm, perceptive mind. It is to experience the merging of all aspects of ourselves — body, mind, and spirit — by learning how to attune to prana and listen to the wisdom of the healer within us.

# Living the Principle of Prana

*When the inner life energy, the prana, begins to become active through the practice of holistic techniques, a unique phenomenon occurs. Our own vital energy, the innate intelligent force within us, begins to correct physiological and psychological blocks lodged within the system. We begin to establish a direct form of communication with the healing force within us. We tap our true nature.*

Yogi Amrit Desai

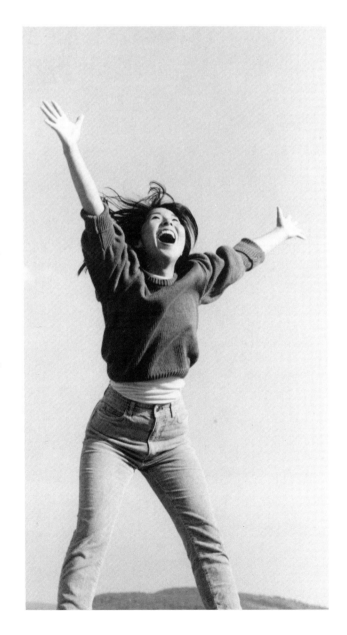

The communication that Yogi Desai speaks of is the reestablishment of contact with our intuition, our inner knowledge of what is right for us as whole, integrated beings. By progressively allowing the evolutionary force of prana to guide us, we have the potential to reach the apex of our energy, a transcendence of normal well-being.

The chart entitled "Levels of Health" symbolizes our growth, through prana, toward true well-being. Health is not holistic unless it encompasses an ascent toward the realm of self-realization. The chart portrays the significance of this definition of health. At its lowest level, health is simply a matter of avoiding death and moving toward a "normal" combination of sickness and health. The focus is mainly on the physical body.

Rising above that level of defining health is the experience of well-being due to harmonious mind-body integration. The orientation is important here, for health now becomes an affirmation rather than an avoidance, a moving toward rather than a flight from.

The Kripalu Approach recognizes the possibility of an even higher level of health and a heightened experience of well-being. Here the focus is on prana, the inner life force, and its potential not only to harmonize body and mind, but to guide us to its most subtle expression within us, that of spirit.

Now there is not only the affirmation of life, but the truest experience and celebration of our inherent potential for wholeness and holiness. For if we follow the continuum of prana, we begin to experience the infinite, sublime seed of life within us. Such an orientation to health holds profound implications for how we live life and the fundamental attitudes we hold toward it.

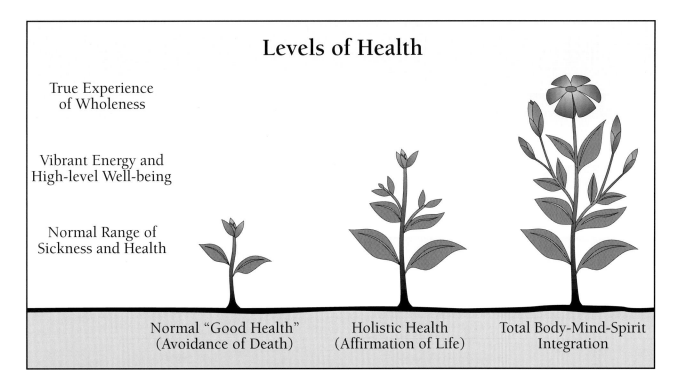

# Levels of Health

True Experience
of Wholeness

Vibrant Energy and
High-level Well-being

Normal Range of
Sickness and Health

Normal "Good Health"
(Avoidance of Death)

Holistic Health
(Affirmation of Life)

Total Body-Mind-Spirit
Integration

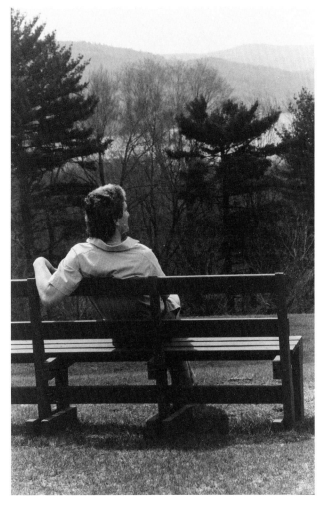

## Where Am I Right Now?

The first step on the Kripalu path to holistic health is
to establish where you are now. The next section of
this book is a specially developed Holistic Health
Appraisal Checklist that will help you draw a baseline from which you can measure your needs and
your progress. By completing it before you read on,
you will experience greater benefits from the chap-
ters that follow.

# Self-Discovery Experience 1

## Checking out your holistic health quotient

The following questionnaire has two main purposes:

(1) to provide you with insights into your current holistic health quotient, which will be a basis for understanding and practicing the methods suggested in this book; and

(2) to provide a baseline against which you can check your progress after you have implemented the techniques of the Kripalu Approach in your daily life for a period of time.

The questionnaire has been constructed in such a way that you can complete it repeatedly, recording your score about every three to six months to see where you've improved.

**NOTE:**
It is important to answer the questions objectively, recording what you really do, not what you would *like to think* you do! Circle the number that corresponds most closely to what you do.

## % of Time

**1. Relaxation**
 a. I am generally relaxed and unworried.
 b. I sleep well and regularly.
 c. I fall asleep easily without help.
 d. I have no trouble getting up.
 e. I take a brief relaxation/meditation daily.

**2. Body**
 a. I feel fit, energetic, and healthy.
 b. I take responsibility for illness.
 c. My body feels flexible and youthful.
 d. My weight and muscle tone are good.

**3. Exercise**
 a. I do vigorous exercise (jog, play tennis, etc.) often (three or more times a week).
 b. I do stretching, limbering, and yoga daily.
 c. I dance or express myself through my body.
 d. I work at improving my fitness.
 e. I walk rather than drive whenever I can.

**4. Leisure/Fun**
 a. I have energy to use my free time creatively.
 b. I feel free to simply have fun without a purpose.
 c. I laugh freely and frequently.
 d. It's easy for me to joke with others.
 e. I don't take life too seriously.

**5. Work**
 a. I enjoy my work to the fullest.
 b. I feel fulfilled and appreciated.
 c. I work a moderate number of hours, avoiding excess overtime.
 d. My communications with co-workers are open and harmonious.
 e. I experience little anxiety, insecurity, or competitiveness.

**6. Diet**
 a. I eat natural, wholesome foods without additives.
 b. I avoid "junk" foods such as soft drinks and chocolate bars.
 c. I eat knowing that food affects my consciousness.
 d. I fast/follow a purification diet at regular intervals.
 e. I avoid stimulants such as coffee, alcohol, colas, and cigarettes.

**7. Communication/Self Expression**
 a. I communicate easily and openly with others.
 b. I am comfortable with new people and groups.
 c. I am a good listener.
 d. I feel free to ask when I need love or caring.
 e. I deal well with my own and other people's emotions.

| 80-100% | 60-80% | 40-60% | 20-40% | 0-20% |
|---|---|---|---|---|

| 80-100% | 60-80% | 40-60% | 20-40% | 0-20% |
|---|---|---|---|---|
| 5 5 5 5 5 | 4 4 4 4 | 3 3 3 3 3 | 2 2 2 2 2 | 1 1 1 1 |
| 5 5 5 5 | 4 4 4 4 | 3 3 3 | 2 2 2 2 | 1 1 1 |
| 5 5 5 5 5 | 4 4 4 4 | 3 3 3 3 | 2 2 2 2 | 1 1 1 1 |
| 5 5 5 5 5 | 4 4 4 4 | 3 3 3 3 | 2 2 2 2 | 1 1 1 1 |
| 5 5 5 5 5 | 4 4 4 4 4 | 3 3 3 3 3 | 2 2 2 2 2 | 1 1 1 1 1 |
| 5 5 5 5 5 | 4 4 4 4 | 3 3 3 3 | 2 2 2 2 | 1 1 1 1 1 |
| 5 5 5 5 5 | 4 4 4 4 4 | 3 3 3 3 3 | 2 2 2 2 2 | 1 1 1 1 1 |

⟹

# Self-Discovery Experience

# 1

# Continued

## Checking out your holistic health quotient

8. *Spirituality/Meditation*
   a. Spirituality plays a role in my life.
   b. I meditate or spend time in introspection.
   c. I meet regularly with others for inspiration.
   d. I express my spirituality in song and music.
   e. I use prayer/affirmation as a healing tool.

9. *Lifestyle/Environment*
   a. My lifestyle supports my health and spiritual needs.
   b. The people I spend my time with are kindred spirits and help me grow.
   c. I do everything in my power to foster my own health and well-being.
   d. I am always seeking new ways to grow.
   e. My family life is peaceful and harmonious.

## Bonus Points

From the following statements, pick the one that comes closest to describing your predominant feeling as you were filling out this questionnaire. Since you are unique, none will exactly describe your feelings, so just pick the one that is closest.

a. I expect I'll get a really high score, because I know I'm doing all I can. I can't wait to see the result.          ( )

b. I'll probably score well in some areas and poorly in others, and that's okay. It'll be interesting and I'll learn about myself.          ( )

c. I hope I'll score well. I don't want to find out I'm not as healthy as I think I am.   ( )

d. I don't suppose I'll score very well. I know I should be doing much more for myself.   ( )

e. Oh dear, I bet I'll get a really low score and then I'll feel awful about myself. Perhaps I won't fill it out.          ( )

There are two things to understand in evaluating your score:

1. *Only you can evaluate your score.* We are not going to give you a range of numbers and tell you a certain score is good or bad. This isn't like any other test you've ever taken because there is no passing mark or norm against which to evaluate yourself and no expectation for you to meet. The whole point of the quiz is for you to see yourself more clearly so you can decide what the implications are for you personally.

   Why are there numbers? So that you can use this quiz to monitor your progress as you implement the methods outlined in this book. If you score yourself each time, it is easier for you to see where you have made significant improvement. The only important function of the numbers is for you to compare yourself to yourself over time — say every three or six months. Here are some suggestions for understanding the meaning of your first non-evaluative score. Ask yourself:

| 80-100% | 60-80% | 40-60% | 20-40% | 0-20% |
|---------|--------|--------|--------|-------|
| 5 | 4 | 3 | 2 | 1 |
| 5 | 4 | 3 | 2 | 1 |
| 5 | 4 | 3 | 2 | 1 |
| 5 | 4 | 3 | 2 | 1 |
| 5 | 4 | 3 | 2 | 1 |

| 80-100% | 60-80% | 40-60% | 20-40% | 0-20% |
|---------|--------|--------|--------|-------|
| 5 | 4 | 3 | 2 | 1 |
| 5 | 4 | 3 | 2 | 1 |
| 5 | 4 | 3 | 2 | 1 |
| 5 | 4 | 3 | 2 | 1 |
| 5 | 4 | 3 | 2 | 1 |

## How to evaluate your score

- Am I satisfied with what I see, in terms of overall results?
- In terms of each individual section?
- Does this tell me that I am as healthy as I can reasonably expect to be at this stage in my life?
- Is my level of health and fitness normal for my age?
- Do I want something more than health and fitness?
- Am I doing the most that I reasonably can to nurture my health?
- What more could/would I like to do?
- How much of a priority is this for me?
- What stands in my way?
- How can I use these answers to help me get more out of this book?
- Which areas am I strong in, and where do I have the potential for improvement?

2. *Your attitude is more important than your score* The last question may have clued you in to that. It is much more important to have a healthy, positive attitude toward your health than to get a high score in the quiz. The questions were developed to help you see where you are right now and where you have the potential to improve. They were not developed to make you feel guilty for all the things you are not doing "right" or "should" be doing differently.

If there were a score, we'd tell you to deduct at least fifty points if you felt guilty, self-rejecting, or "bad" when you filled out the questionnaire! The best way to interpret your findings is with objectivity and lack of emotion, to the extent that you are able. It seems to be a natural human tendency to see our inadequacies more clearly than the things we are doing right.

So look at your answers in this spirit: "Some things I'm doing at the level I'd like to; some are areas that I haven't developed yet in myself. That's exciting because learning is always interesting, especially learning about myself. Who said I had to be perfect, anyway?"

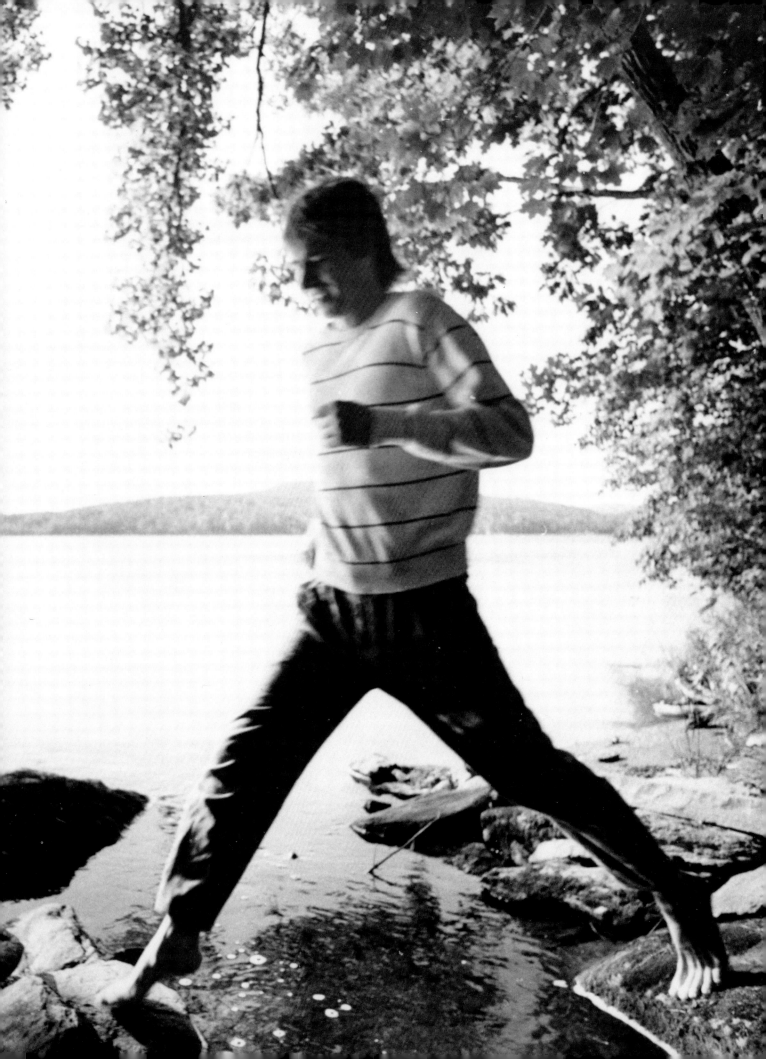

# *The Journey*

## how do I get there from here?

# The Kripalu Approach:
# The Eight Pathways to Health

The Kripalu Approach to health and high level well-being is a combination of holistic health techniques from East and West. It is organized into eight pathways based on the eight major ways in which we express our energy in day-to-day living:

1. Living a More Relaxed Life
2. Getting to Know and Love Your Body
3. Learning How to Play
4. Learning the Art of Relaxed Work
5. Discovering Your Optimum Diet
6. Mastering Communication — with Yourself and Others
7. Practicing Meditation and Spiritual Attunement
8. Creating a Supportive Lifestyle

The above ways of expressing reflect what you might do in any twenty-four hour day to maintain your life's activities and relationships. Each plays a significant and equal role as a means through which you interact with the prana energy within you.

The Kripalu Approach uses natural tools from modern and ancient traditions of healing to harmonize the energy in each area. Once you are on your way to a harmony of being that embraces how you eat, sleep, work, and play, you enter a realm of health beyond your present experience.

This approach to holistic health is very practical. Guests tell us that practicing a daily schedule at Kripalu that includes yoga, relaxation, play, and proper diet gives them an opportunity to establish positive health habits. They say that the tools they learn, which are the same as those in this Guide, help them create when they return home a lifestyle that is more harmonious and more supportive of their aspirations for perfect health.

Lifestyle is the keystone of holistic health. Our present state of incomplete health and happiness is the result of choices we have made, consciously or unconsciously, in all areas of our lives. Now we are taking responsibility to make new choices, to make changes. That requires energy and effort, and it is made easier if we accept the fact that habit patterns cannot be changed overnight. The ability to maintain an attitude of flexibility and patience while working at making changes is essential.

Qualities of self-acceptance, patience, and sincerity are hallmarks of the healthy person. Those qualities will aid you in using this book to walk toward health, enjoying in each moment of the journey the pleasure of your own company, your body, mind, and spirit, as you begin to experience the radiant energy of prana that is your birthright.

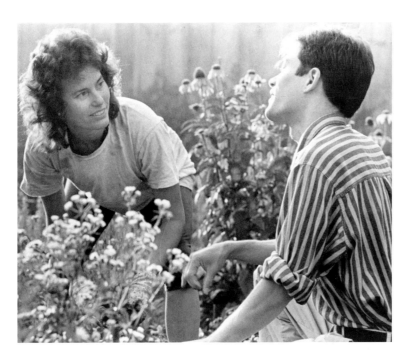

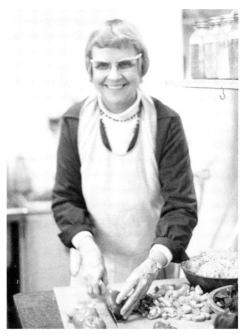

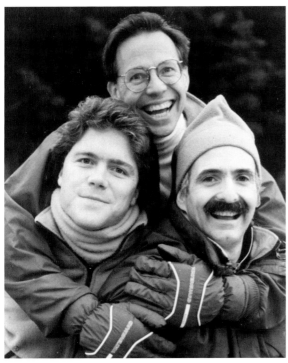

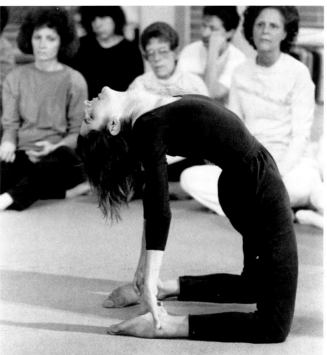

# THE FOUR VOICES OF PRANA
## by Yogi Amrit Desai

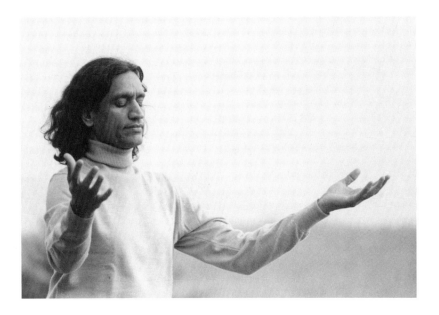

The Kripalu approach to holistic health is based on our becoming reattuned to prana, that is, learning to live again in the most natural way possible, in accordance with the guidance of our inner life force.

Usually we make choices based on what we think we need or simply on what will satisfy our five senses, rather than on what is good for the health of our bodies. We only hear our minds talking to us, not our bodies. Our goal is to reestablish communication with our prana; to learn to hear and heed its messages again.

One of the most basic levels at which we can reestablish our communication with prana is through the biological urges of the body. Prana communicates these life-giving messages to us privately and personally, sending them to the mind via the nervous system.

Some examples of those kinds of messages are thirst (which is a signal that we need to drink liquids), fatigue, (signaling a need to rest), hunger, tension, and fullness of the bladder or colon. All those messages are a mild form of pain, so mild that we rarely think of them as such. If they are attended to promptly and properly, they immediately turn into the bliss of satisfaction and relief.

When we respond to the messages appropriately, we reap increased physical health, vitality, and mental peace. When we ignore, resist, or postpone responding, prana's messages become more pronounced and urgent.

Prana communicates its signals to the mind in four stages of increasing intensity. Knowledge of these stages will make it easier for you to attune your mind to prana and to harmonize your daily activities to this inner wisdom. The aligning of your activities to prana will help you create greater holistic health and avoid premature degeneration and aging of your body.

## Stage One: Cooperation with Prana for Prevention of Disease

In Stage One, prana signals the basic inner needs of our bodies to our minds through the nervous system. The inner signals are experienced as urges, such as the urges to eat, drink, sleep, rest, or eliminate. Those needs must be met if prana is to fulfill its primary function of body maintenance, protection, and healing. The function of the mind at this stage is to cooperate with prana by locating and securing from the external world whatever prana needs to sustain the body and keep it healthy.

In this first stage, prana is under the control of the mind. This is a crucial stage, where the mind can either choose to assist and support the involuntary functions of the body by responding to prana's signals, or ignore the signals and disrupt the natural, involuntary functions of the body. For the mind to respond to the inner urges of the body and carry them out appropriately is an act of prana-mind or body-mind harmony.

If the mind, however, turns its back on prana's signals and chooses to fulfill the ego's desires, dreams, fears, and fantasies, it will automatically be in conflict with the body. Such conflicts of mind with the universal laws of prana lead to physical tension, mental restlessness, and strain. If we do not change the orientation of our minds from the desires of the ego back to prana we are eventually headed for trouble in the form of more serious physical and mental disorders.

During the first stage, the role of the mind is extremely important. If our mind is calm and clear, we will choose to fulfill the inner needs of the body. If the mind chooses to serve the ego's wants, it will choose a course of action that is not in tune with prana. For example, sometimes we respond to the needs of prana immediately, by resting when we are tired, by eating when we are hungry, or by responding to the urge of elimination promptly. By such appropriate responses, we keep our energy high and insure good physical health.

At other times however, we may delay or resist responding to prana's signals and, as a result, our store of energy is depleted and our body suffers unnecessary wear and tear. Often we respond to the needs of prana only partially, such as by eating promptly when we are hungry, yet eating foods that emphasize taste rather than nourishment.

Sometimes we ignore prana because of peer pressure, which might cause us to stay late at a party when our inner voice is telling us to go home to bed, or because of social customs, which might lead us to wear constricting clothing that we know our bodies are not comfortable in. Sometimes we may tune out the inner messages of prana to follow guidance from outside that may not be at all suited to our individual needs, such as the latest health fads or diet theories. In this first stage, we have that choice; how we choose determines the intensity of prana's next message to us.

## Stage Two:
## The Early Warning Signals of Sickness

In this stage, short-term pain prompts action, although there is still some choice. If our mind has ignored prana's signals and not responded to the needs of the body in Stage One, prana must correct the imbalance that we have created. Because the neglected need is causing increasing wear and tear on the body, prana is now forced to escalate the intensity of its messages to the mind in the form of greater pain, distress, tension, or strain.

The pain is only of sufficient intensity to become noticeable to the mind that has successfully ignored the signals of the previous stage. For example, if we ignore prana's signal to empty our bladder when we get the first signal of slight discomfort, that discomfort eventually intensifies so much that we must pay attention to it. Or if we postpone responding to prana's signal of tiredness, which tells us to quit work for the

day, prana will increase the intensity of the message by signaling the need to rest with a headache or backache, or fatigue, eyestrain, or irritability.

Those kinds of signals are prana's method of getting our attention and letting us know that we are mistreating our bodies in some way. During this warning stage the messages from prana may be only occasional mild pain or fatigue, or minor physical disorders such as colds, indigestion, or slightly elevated blood pressure. Accompanying the physical complaints may be mental tension, irritability, or minor emotional disturbances.

If we respond to the messages of Stage Two, prana can correct the imbalances we have created in a short time and with a minimum of strain on our bodies. Occasional discomfort or pain is the price we pay for ignoring the signals of the first stage and to restore the bodily imbalances we have created. If we ignore this pain or suppress it with tranquilizers, antacids, aspirin, or other medication and continue to put excessive strain on the body, the body will begin to deteriorate further.

At this stage we may be tempted to treat the symptoms in such a way as to achieve immediate relief, rather than going to the real cause of the problem. The earlier we respond appropriately to bodily needs, the less effort it takes to rectify the imbalance and the greater will be the results of our effort. Prevention is always better than cure.

## Stage Three: Time to Look for a Cure

In this stage, fear of long-term pain and disability virtually forces us to act. As explained in Stage Two, if we fail to respond to prana's warnings and continue to treat our bodies with the same lack of consciousness, prana must resort to stronger, more obvious signals to draw the attention of our restless minds to the damage we are doing.

During this stage, prana sends signals of intense pain to warn us that various problems are now beginning to develop. Serious disorders and diseases that are starting to manifest in our bodies as pain are prana's cry for urgent attention.

What was indigestion in Stage Two has now become signs of a peptic ulcer. Moderately high blood pressure has developed into symptoms of cardiac insufficiency, angina pectoris, or a mild heart attack. Morning stiffness in the joints has become the pains of arthritis. Our condition now demands medical attention.

The signals of prana during this stage are usually strong enough to force even those who are out of touch with their bodies to seek medical aid. Our bodies are now incapacitated for significant periods of time and we become fearful over our state of health.

We rarely have much energy, for prana is mainly occupied with constantly repairing the accumulated damage as well as the damage we are continuing to inflict. The state of low energy makes us less efficient at our day-to-day responsibilities. Our inefficiency makes us tense and, as a result, we become even less efficient and more fearful. That becomes a constant drain on our physical, mental, emotional, and financial resources, and we may begin to develop psychological problems such as chronic anxiety or depression.

For treatment to be successful at this stage we must seek professional assistance, change our life style, and practice attending to our bodily needs. Now we must attend to that which we ignored in Stage One, but with more pain, more effort, and less effectiveness. If these two regimens — external and internal change — are not followed conscientiously and wholeheartedly, our physical condition will deteriorate into Stage Four.

## Stage Four: Incapacitating and Life-Threatening Illness

Fear of death controls our actions in this stage, and we have no choice whether to respond or not. If we have not changed our lifestyle as indicated in Stage Three, but have continued to overstrain our bodies, the condition of our affected bodily organs and systems will continue to deteriorate. Prana now steps up the intensity of its signals to Stage Four.

In this stage, self-cure is almost impossible and we experience a critical breakdown of organs or systems in our bodies, requiring immediate, often radical, medical intervention in the form of hospitalization, major surgery, intensive care, and/or prolonged convalescence. Often there is long-term physical disability that can make it difficult or impossible for us to provide for our own needs or continue to support a family.

# Mind and Prana — A Tragicomedy in Pictures

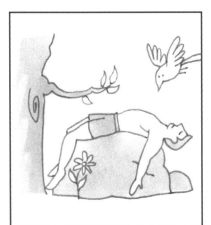

*In the beginning, the body was limp and lifeless until…*

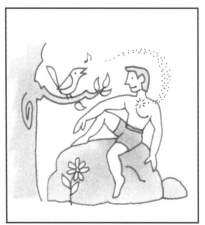

*Prana, the life force, joined the body and gave him life!*

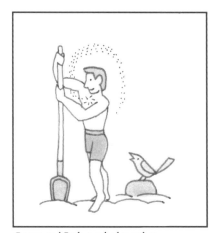

*Prana and Body worked together…*

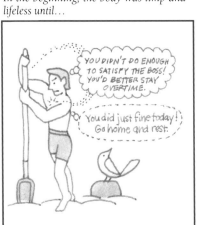

*At work a similar thing happened. Body worked all day very efficiently. When it was time to go, Prana was satisfied and ready to quit. But Mind had other ideas….*

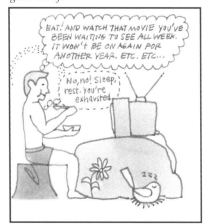

*After pushing into overtime at work, Body is exhausted. After being ignored all day, Prana's voice is weaker and makes very little impression on the mind.*

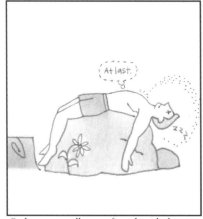

*Body, now totally out of touch with the voice of Prana, collapses.*

Some of the physiological and psychological conditions that are typical of Stage Four are stroke with partial paralysis, perforated ulcer necessitating removal of part of the digestive system, acute psychosis or suicidal depression requiring hospitalization, massive heart attack, and cancer.

Now prana's ability to work freely to accomplish healing is so inhibited by the physical and emotional blocks we have accumulated that it can't recover easily to heal the body or mind's condition. It is barely able to drive the most vital organs and systems to keep the body clinically alive.

Only when the mind has failed to accept — because of its preoccupations, conditioning, and distractions — all the accumulated violations of prana in the previous stages, does prana resort to the intense signals of Stage Four. Now the signals dramatically and urgently present to the mind the necessity of paying attention to the body if the body is going to survive. Thus, prana upgrades the intensity of its signals in each successive stage only enough to capture the attention of the mind and no more.

All stages of physical distress, from mere discomfort through severe pain, are simply messengers of prana with a single, simple purpose: to show us where we are going astray on the road of life and health, and to bring us back. They are like welcome lighthouses glimpsed through the fog, warning us to take our bearing and correct our course before we steer onto the rocks.

Once we understand that, a change will happen in our attitude toward pain and sickness, health, and life itself. We will become willing and able to respond to the warning signals that prana sends us in the earliest stage, and so lead a life of prevention rather than cure, a life that is full of the joy and freedom of holistic health.

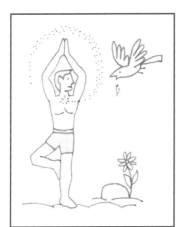

they played together....

*Prana and Body worked together in perfect harmony. They listened to each other's needs very attentively. Whenever Prana needed to eat, Body ate. Whenever Prana wanted to sleep, Body slept.... Thus Body and Prana lived in harmony, complete in themselves, happy and healthy. Pure mind observed, enjoyed, and supported the natural friendship of Body and Prana.*

*Then one day, Mind discovered dreaming and scheming...wanting to be the boss ... It had many desires... So Mind began to manipulate to receive the things it wanted, in the way it wanted.*

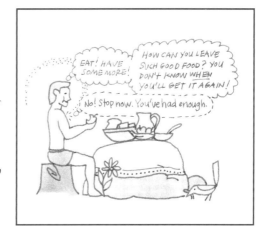

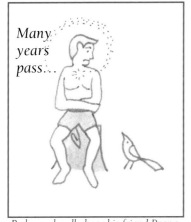

Body can hardly hear his friend Prana anymore, which is pleading with him to stop.

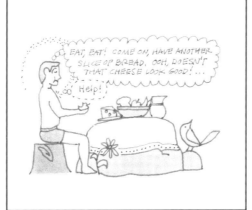

After Body has been enslaved to Mind, he is in poor physical, mental, and emotional shape. What can Body do? One good look in the mirror says enough.

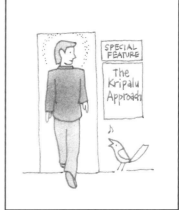

Yet Body needn't despair. There is a way to return to that natural state of balance between the body and the mind....

# Self-Discovery Experience 2

## Testing your ability to listen to prana

Now draw on your own experience for a more in-depth understanding of the principles we've discussed. First find a quiet place to complete this introspection. Then close your eyes for a moment and think of a situation where you felt conflicting urges. Adjacent are some examples to get you started.

As you get in touch with the situation, identify which voice was the voice of prana, your wisdom or real physical need, and which was the voice of the desires stimulated by your mind and senses. Remember what you did and how you felt, physically and mentally, afterward.

Think of several such situations, some where you listened to prana and some where you listened to your mind. You may want to write them down to help you see a pattern.

---

**Example 1**

| | |
|---|---|
| **Prana said:** | "Yawn! I need to go to bed." |
| **Mind said:** | "But I want to watch the Late Late Show. It's especially good tonight." |
| **I did:** | I stayed up. |
| **I felt:** | I felt very tired and irritable the next day. |

---

**Example 2**

| | |
|---|---|
| **Prana said:** | "OK! I've eaten enough. I don't need any more." |
| **Mind said:** | "But this lasagna's so delicious. And who knows when I'll be able to have some again?" |
| **I did:** | I ate it. |
| **I felt:** | I felt too full, sluggish, and upset, and had to take an Alka Seltzer. |

## Example 4

| | |
|---|---|
| **Prana said:** | "Get up and go jogging; you'll feel great afterward." |
| **Mind said:** | "But I'm so warm and comfortable and sleepy. I must need the extra rest." |
| **I did:** | I stayed in bed. |
| **I felt:** | I felt half-awake all morning because I slept too long and didn't get enough exercise. |

## Example 3

| | |
|---|---|
| **Prana said:** | "This room is so stuffy and I'm stiff from sitting here all day. I need some fresh air and exercise." |
| **Mind said:** | "But I want to get this project finished so I'll get praise when the boss comes." |
| **I did:** | I took a short, brisk walk. |
| **I felt:** | I felt revived and I finished the project anyway because I was more alert. |

## Example 5

| | |
|---|---|
| **Prana said:** | "You'd better not combine those two foods. You know they'll upset your digestion." |
| **Mind said:** | "It won't hurt just this once." |
| **I did:** | I saved one for later. |
| **I felt:** | I felt good, no indigestion. |

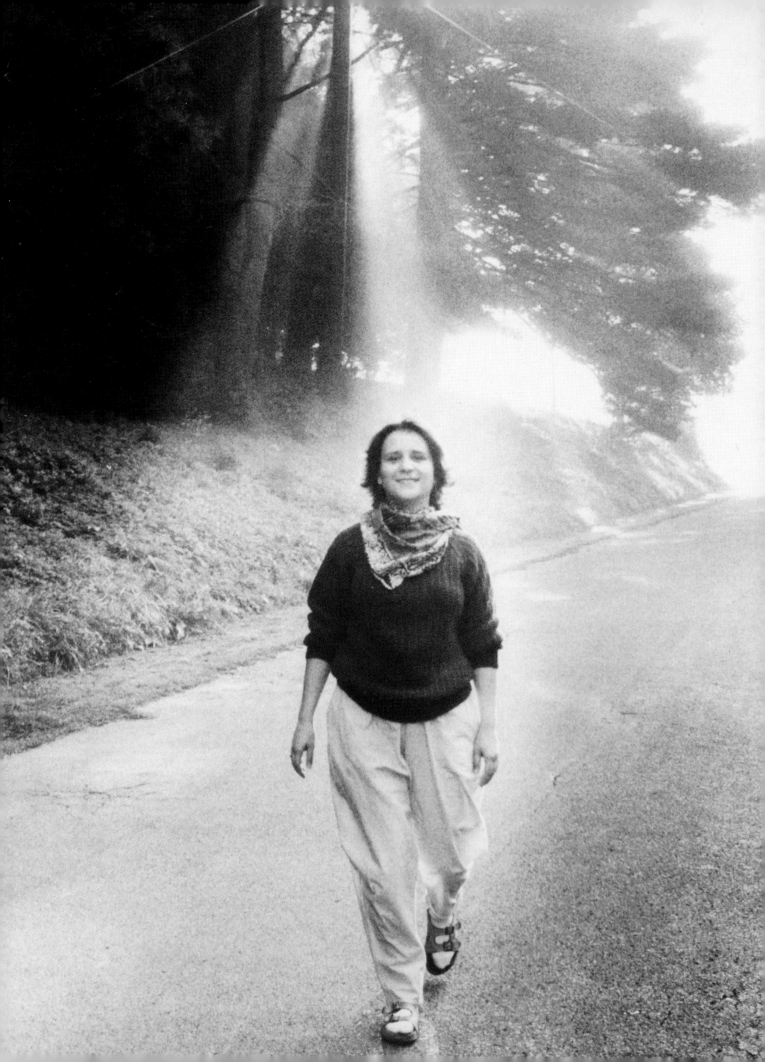

# The First Pathway

living a more relaxed life

# Relaxation Is an Attitude

Each time you feel tension it tells you there is something that needs attention. Tension is the result of our lifestyle, our past, or our expectations. It acts as a block between us and the universal energy of prana. When we relax we become like a sponge and draw in the pranic energy of our surroundings.

In the midst of our busy lives it's easy to forget that rest and relaxation are as crucial to our well-being as the air we breathe or the food we eat. Throughout the night, as we rest in the deepest of relaxations, nature (prana) proceeds to heal us while the mind remains quiet and the body still. The same deep healing can occur in the wakeful state, but many of us seem to have lost touch with the natural state of relaxation.

The articles that follow present a detailed, practical understanding of stress, tension, and relaxation. They express a philosophy that has two fundamental principles: one, that stress is not necessarily bad and does not automatically lead to the experience of tension; and two, that relaxation is much more than what you need when you are feeling tense or what you do when you are not doing anything else.

Relaxation, in the Kripalu Approach, is an attitude to life that can be cultivated. It is a way of living, a state to be experienced in each moment, no matter what you may be doing. If you can learn to live that way, you will prevent or greatly diminish the accumulation of tension that has been proven to cause most of our prevalent diseases.

This chapter also includes some easy-to-follow exercises that will help you to identify what causes you, personally, to experience tension, whether mental or physical, and how to go about relaxing those specific tensions.

The First Pathway is at top right.

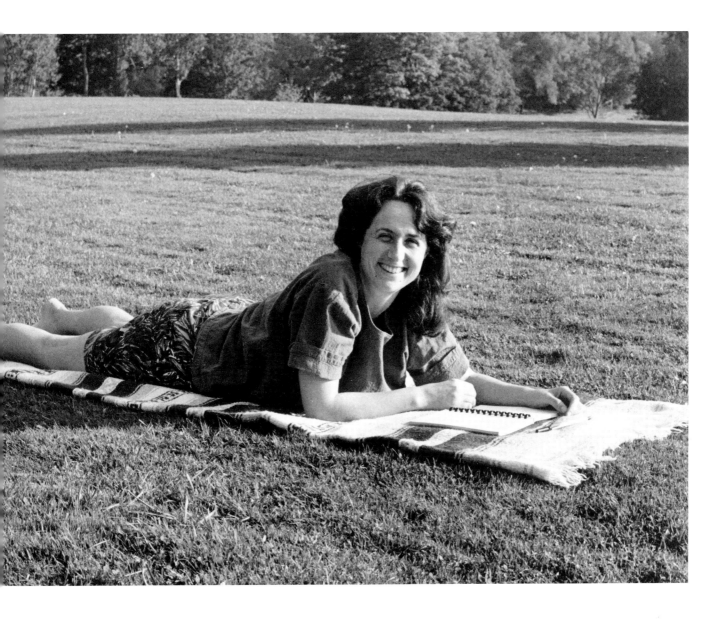

## Redefining Stress

What does the word *stress* evoke for you? Pressure perhaps, fearful situations, difficulty in relationships, accident and injury, demands and expectations, feeling inadequate? Those are responses that came to people's minds when they were asked that question. What would you add to the list?

Interestingly, those are all situations with negative or undesirable connotations. Yet in his book *Stress Without Distress*, Dr. Hans Selye defines stress as a neutral physiological phenomenon, devoid of any value connotations of desirable or undesirable. In his view, stress is a "non-specific response of the body to any demand made on it."

Only after we have experienced the initial physiological reaction to the external situation does our conscious mind interpret the experience as positive or negative. So our association of stress with only undesirable phenomena is a one-sided definition.

Consequently, the first thing to understand about stress is that it is a neutral, natural, and normal response of the body to any external situation that places a demand on the body's energy resources. Pleasure, joy, happiness, and excitement also elicit the body's stress response, but since we do not see them as undesirable or seek to avoid them, the energy drain is less and we do not experience those emotions as stressful.

Stress is not only a normal reaction of the body, but also one that is necessary to the maintenance of our lives. Responding to stress enables us to take the actions necessary to keep ourselves alive, free from danger, and evolving as a species.

How then has stress become such a negative concept in present day society? Eighty percent of illnesses are said to be caused by stress, and "stress management," "deep relaxation," and "tension release" are sought after by everyone. Why the tension headaches, the ulcers, the whole range of stress-related ailments if stress is a neutral, normal, and natural part of being alive?

Stress is considered negative because we have not consciously examined and understood the ancient, instinctual, physiological stress pattern. We have not realized that we are still responding to stress at the same instinctual level as our ancestors. Their stress response was appropriate to them: life was precarious and the ones who survived to propagate the species were those who were fastest, strongest, and fiercest in the face of the life-threatening situations that occurred daily.

When they sensed danger, the autonomic (instinctual) nervous system signaled the body to release the hormone adrenaline into the blood stream, providing instant energy to the heart, lungs, and muscles to adapt and adjust the organism for "fight or flight." Our bodies still respond with this same ancient mechanism that rushes intense energy to us for fight or flight.

But our lives have changed. As we have evolved as a species, our new interpretations of the events around us have been intermingled and confused with our instinctual unconscious reactions. As a result, we do not cope effectively with stress and we experience tension. We need to start our process of learning to relax by making an important distinction between stress and tension. Stress is a natural, physiological phenomenon necessary to life. Tension is the unpleasant physical and mental repercussion we experience when we are not able to process our stress effectively.

## From Stress to Tension

How does stress become tension? First, it is a result of our unconsciously continued habit of perceiving unexpected external situations as threatening, when in reality they need not be. In present-day society, trust, cooperation, and interaction could be our mode of interaction. Yet jungle law still prevails in our minds, so "survival of the fittest" is still our unconscious law of life.

If we overhear criticism of a task we have performed, we often respond with fear and anger as if it were a threat to our very life, rather than simply an evaluation of an action we happened to do less well than was expected. Our "survival of the fittest" internal mechanical programming says "Defend yourself, or you will die!" and we experience fear, as if our very life were threatened. That is our first mistake.

The second way we set ourselves up to experience tension is our lack of awareness of our physiological processes. We don't realize until too late that our unnecessary fears are generating a chain of physiological reactions, such as the adrenaline secretion that causes the rush of energy to muscles and heart for fight or flight. All of a sudden our heart is thumping, we feel restless energy, and we start to experience a need to express it through anger or through vigorously defending ourselves.

Because we do not consciously experience our negative emotions simply as energy coupled with inappropriate thinking patterns, we repress them as bad or antisocial. Our unexpressed energy is then experienced as physical tension: step three on our journey from neutral stress to negative tension.

Another cause of tension is using mental energy to fight something we cannot physically control or change. For instance, if I am sitting in heavy traffic, not moving, and I know I am going to be late for an important meeting, I have two choices. I can fume and rage and be frustrated at the unplanned, uncontrollable, and unnecessary delay: "Why don't they do something about this bottleneck?" "Why don't people go home earlier, a different way?" "It's so stupid!" Or I can sit back, relax, and accept the inevitable. It's clear that I will feel much more tense and drained by the first response than the second one, yet most of us respond in the first way.

When tensions accumulate, we feel a discomfort that we try either to ignore or to release in inappropriate ways, such as using alcohol, food, drugs, or sex. Unfortunately, our nonacceptance of our basic physical-emotional experience is a further cause of tension. The more tense we become, the more we lose energy; the lower our energy, the more prone we are to perceive neutral events as threats, to experience fear, and to start the cycle over again. So tension is a downward spiral, fueled by fear and lack of conscious understanding.

Tension is not inherent in a situation or caused by someone else. Although, at our present point in history, we are probably surrounded by more potentially tension-creating situations than ever before, we can learn to respond to those situations without tension. Evidence abounds for that all around us, but we do not always see it clearly.

The same situation can make one person extremely tense, angry, or fearful, while someone else is able to remain relatively relaxed and unconcerned. For instance, I may experience a visit to the dentist as extremely stressful and become very tense. You may remain completely relaxed and joke your way through the experience.

We are all the end products of very different programming, so what evokes fear in one person does not press another's panic button. And some of us simply seem to have had more fear programmed into us.

## Two Ways to Break the Tension Cycle: Physical and Mental

What is the solution? How can we break the tension cycle and learn to be more relaxed, happy human beings? That is what the Kripalu Approach is about. It teaches that we can intervene in the cycle at every stage in the process on two different levels: physical and mental.

On the physical level, we can practice many different relaxation techniques that will raise and balance our energy and make us less prone to experience events and people as threatening. Since breath is the link between mind, body, and emotions, we can learn to intervene in and override the physiological fight-or-flight response through special breathing exercises, two of which are detailed in the next chapter, "The Second Pathway."

On the mental level, we can intervene by accepting responsibility for our evolution as conscious beings and refusing to continue responding mechanically and instinctively as if every unexpected and undesired event were a survival-level threat. We can observe

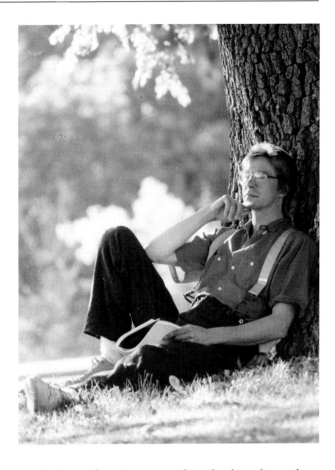

our feelings of tension, trace them back to the underlying fear or imagined threat, and see that it was not in fact a threat to our survival, but merely to our pride, our security, or our superficial ego.

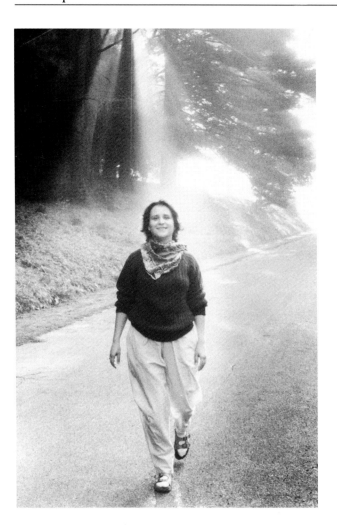

That kind of mental stance means learning to re-interpret our world and changing some of the attitudes we believe are part of us and with which we feel secure. As a wise man has said, "We must, at every moment, be prepared to give up what we are for what we can become."

Living a relaxed life begins to happen as we consciously develop new adaptive processes for dealing with stress in our lives. We can cultivate an alternative to the fight-or-flight response: acceptance of and cooperation with whatever situations life sends our way. Tension will then diminish little by little until it becomes a thing of the past.

The exercises and articles that follow have been structured to help you become more familiar with how you convert stress into tension. They also provide many concrete, practical techniques both for overcoming your stress response in specific kinds of situations and for leading a more relaxed life in general.

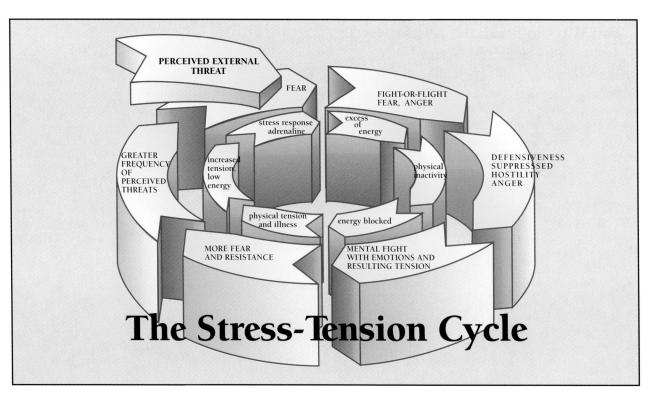

# The Stress-Tension Cycle

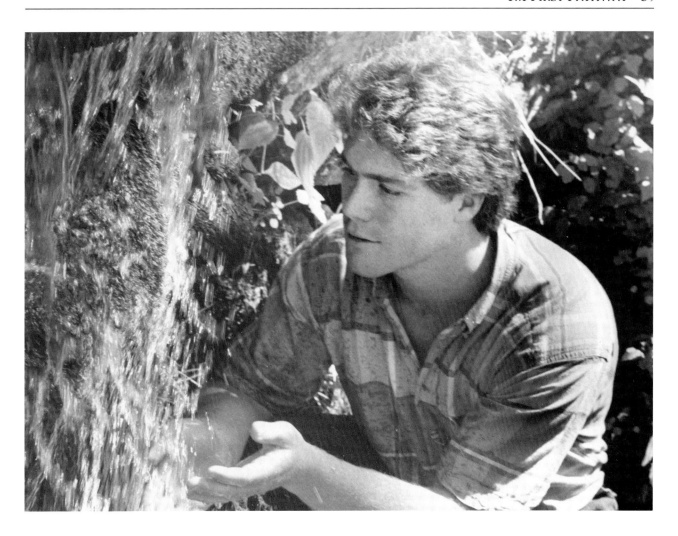

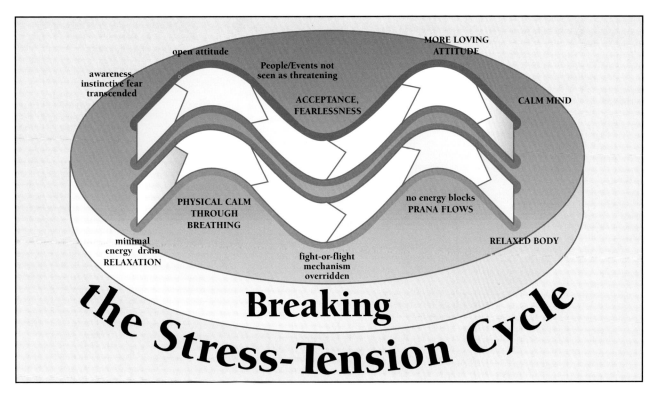

**Breaking the Stress-Tension Cycle**

open attitude

awareness, instinctive fear transcended

People/Events not seen as threatening

ACCEPTANCE, FEARLESSNESS

MORE LOVING ATTITUDE

CALM MIND

PHYSICAL CALM THROUGH BREATHING

no energy blocks PRANA FLOWS

minimal energy drain RELAXATION

fight-or-flight mechanism overridden

RELAXED BODY

# Self-Discovery Experience 3

## Fight or flight — what are your hidden stress patterns?

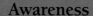

Becoming aware of what causes you to experience tension — when, where, and why — is the key to learning to deal with it.

**DIRECTIONS:** Choose a quiet place to sit where you can complete this introspection without interruption. After reading each question, close your eyes, take some slow deep breaths to relax your body and calm your mind, then begin to let the thoughts, images, and associations flow.

1.  Reflect on a recent situation in which you were conscious of experiencing tension in the form of impatience, fear, anger, irritation, guilt, or blame. Allow yourself to relive that situation in your mind's eye. See clearly the person(s) involved and reexperience the thoughts that came. Let the emotions flow over you, as if it were happening now. In this setting, you don't have to control or hide your feelings for social reasons, so just let them envelop you. Sink into them without judgement or rationalization.

2.  After a few minutes, notice what is happening to you physiologically. Has your breathing changed? Do you feel hot or cold? Is any part of your body tense (tight jaw, clenched fist, tight abdomen, frown?) What are your thoughts? Are they clear and objective, or confused and blurred?

3.  Ask yourself: "How do I feel about the person(s) involved? Can I clearly see a solution? What is it I wanted and didn't get? Do I know exactly what to do next to remove the stress? What do I want to do, right now, to feel better?" When these answers are clear to you, slowly open your eyes and write them down.

    (a) Physically, I felt/noticed . . .

    (b) My thoughts were . . .

    (c) About the person(s) involved, I felt . . .

    (d) I wanted to feel better by . . .

    (e) In this situation, what I wanted (and didn't get, or thought I wouldn't get) was . . .

4.  Repeat for several situations to get a clearer picture of your reaction patterns.

## Acceptance

5. Review what you have written above and, after reflection, complete these sentences honestly, without self-criticism or judgement:
   (a) The kinds of things that make me tense are . . .
   (b) When I become tense, I realize that my body responds by . . .
   (c) When I become tense, I notice that my mind and emotions . . .
   (d) When I become tense, I want to remove that feeling and feel better by . . .
   (e) What I generally want from situations that cause me stress is . . .

## Adjustment

### How to Transform Your Tension Reaction into a Relaxation Response

Now that you understand more clearly how your tensions are caused, you can begin to find ways to relax in those situations:

6. Begin to observe yourself day to day so that you are able to see tension approaching from a distance or catch it happening. Then accept it! If you fight it or try to suppress it or get angry at yourself for reacting to it, you'll get more tense and lose more energy. Just recognize it and allow yourself to feel the symptoms in your body.

7. As tension happens, consciously begin to relax by breathing more slowly and deeply. Your emotions are intimately connected to your breathing patterns (see the section on breathing in "The Second Pathway"). By changing your pattern, you will quickly be able to change any train of thought, even a stressful one. A change in breathing also changes the physical responses that go with emotional or mental tension, such as tightness in the abdomen or shoulders.

   The beauty of it is that deep breathing can be practiced anywhere without anyone even noticing — at work, while traveling, or in a situation of confrontation. So when you feel your body beginning to experience the tension response, immediately begin to take long, deep, regular breaths.

   The natural way of breathing when relaxed is deeply and steadily — just watch a sleeping child or an animal at rest. As you breathe more deeply you will feel refreshed because you are taking in more prana. You will also feel calmer and more objective and able to deal with the situation more efficiently.

8. Recognize whether you are experiencing a fight response or a flight response, and see if you can change your thinking/attitude about the situation. (See the following exercises.)

9. Recognize what you want from the situation and are not getting, and see if you can drop that desire. Accept what is actually happening, rather than trying to fight mentally and emotionally for what you want to have happen.

10. Examine your daily routine to see if you are creating physical situations that predispose you to experience tension. For example, you will be more likely to feel tension if any of the following are true: you are over-tired from lack of sleep; you have overeaten or eaten the wrong kinds of food or too late at night; you have taken too many stimulants, such as coffee, alcohol, or cigarettes; you habitually overwork; you don't get enough play and recreation; or you don't get enough fresh air and exercise.

    See where you can make changes — small ones, one at a time. Don't take on too much! Just regulate your sleep, for instance, or try walking instead of driving once in a while to get more fresh air and exercise.

11. Incorporate some specific physical and mental techniques into your daily schedule, such as hatha yoga, walking, meditation, or sports. Also, take time out to lie down and relax deeply once a day for fifteen to twenty minutes.

# TENSION IS AN ENERGY CRISIS
## by Yogi Amrit Desai

Tension is an energy crisis. It arises from the misuse or abuse of energy. Tension is inefficiency; it is the inability to work at peak performance level. When a car is finely tuned, all of the engine's moving parts work in total harmony with each other. As a result, the car gets the highest possible mileage with the minimum of gasoline. In other words, the output of energy is maximum.

In the same way, each aspect of a person must work in harmony with all other aspects. The body must be healthy, the emotions balanced, and the mind attuned to the body, emotions, and prana. Then our capacity to put forth effort and accomplish work is so high that we get the maximum amount of work done with the minimum expenditure of energy. Harmony of being is the true state of relaxation.

## Seeking Harmony of Being

To create the state of total harmony of being, we must first know what creates the disharmony or tension within us. Tension has two sources: physical disharmony and mental disharmony. Insufficient sleep, insufficient exercise, not eating or digesting properly — those and other unbalanced physical habits can result in physical tension.

Something as simple as posture can be a cause of tension. If we carry our bodies improperly or sit, stand, or walk incorrectly, our bodies will be filled with tension. Each physical habit needs to be taken into consideration in order to effect a permanent change in our ability to relax.

Although tension can have definite physical causes, our mental attitude toward ourselves and our surroundings is the primary source of our disharmony and tension. For example, two of the chief causes of tension are competition and jealousy. When people are motivated to work by those feelings, their purpose is defeated. Instead of gaining from their labor, they lose consistently, because competition and jealousy inevitably lead to fear and insecurity, which in turn give birth to more tension as people feel pressured to work more efficiently at a job they often dislike. The

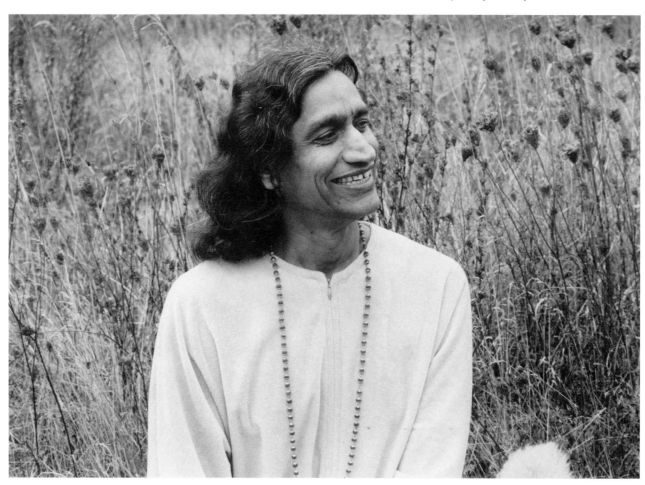

need for efficiency gives birth to still greater tension as they begin to realize their own inadequacies.

Feelings of inadequacy may manifest in either a superiority or an inferiority complex, both of which prevent people from understanding each other. Such misunderstandings again create tension. Thus at every level of activity, many people sink more and more deeply into an unending cycle of tension.

## Living for Today

In order to escape the misunderstandings and feelings of inadequacy that arise in their external situations, these people then seek refuge in their imagination. They live in tomorrow, filled with hopes and desires for the future. The more they desire for the future, the less they are satisfied with today. Their increased dissatisfaction produces greater and greater tension. Then their hopes for tomorrow cause greater incapacity to act efficiently today and they become increasingly more insecure.

To fight this self-produced insecurity, such people strive to pack more and more fun into their day, to consume more, to store more for tomorrow's fun. Their striving creates more insecurity. The frantic fun-seeking, the need to collect and consume for tomorrow, brings many fears. People then have too many choices for today and too many desires for tomorrow. And that makes them restless, insecure, and incapable of enjoying life in the present.

## Warning: Competition May Be Harmful to Your Health

Restlessness prevents such people from finding satisfaction and leads to dissatisfaction in their personal lives and dislike for their work. Dislike for work creates tension which further undermines their efficiency and leads to self-pity, lack of confidence, and a destructive self-image. Those feelings consume a tremendous amount of energy.

Once depleted of energy, people suffer from depression, loneliness, and fear. In order to forget their problems they may resort to drinking, smoking, overeating, excessive sex, drugs, and other forms of escape that either dull or artificially excite their nerves.

To relax they often engage in the competition of games and sports. But even there they do not escape competition, they merely change the arena of competition because their competitive minds are still present. They try painting or golfing or playing chess, but the activity doesn't help them relax because they have not changed their competitive mental attitudes. So long as the newness of the game lasts, they feel that they have changed.

Soon, however, the newness wears off. The habitual attitudes return, and recreation once again is just another source of aggression, fear, fighting, jealousy, and tension. As a result, they end up breaking their golf clubs on the golf course or tearing up their canvas in painting class. They cannot enjoy their work and they no longer know how to play.

If these people continue to resort to escapes and crutches, their escapes become subconscious drives and habits that bring an endless array of physical, mental, and emotional disorders that result from the condition of stress: chronic fatigue, insomnia, restlessness, headaches, stomach ulcers, indigestion, constipation, obesity, and pains in the back and shoulders.

Tension creates all these problems in the first place, and eventually each of these symptoms creates further tension, thus establishing a vicious cycle.

## Finding Inner Balance

The superficial changes to which the average person resorts provide only temporary solutions. The real answer to these problems is to go within and get in touch with one's true inner needs. While there has been astonishing progress made in the material world, most people have failed to adjust their inner lives to keep pace with their mounting external progress and prosperity. As a result, external progress and prosperity have become a burden rather than an asset to peace of mind.

Through the practice of listening to prana, we learn the secrets of balancing body, mind, and inner energies to function effectively amid the pressures of modern society. We learn to hear our inner requests for self-care and nurturance. If we choose to respond, we relieve ourselves of the tension of acting against our natural needs. Instead, we act in harmony with the inner forces of nature or prana, which are always working to establish homeostasis — a balanced, relaxed state of being.

## Self-Discovery Experience

## 4

### How to remove tension by changing your point of view

Since most of our apparent problems come simply from lack of understanding, we can actually dissolve the tension they bring by changing the way we look at them. Resistance to stress — that is, non-acceptance of the inevitable or what is presently happening — causes most tension. We can remove that resistance by a better understanding of our attitudes and transform our stressors by changing how we view them.

**DIRECTIONS:** Use this introspection guide to help you pinpoint attitudes that cause you unnecessary tension and see how to change them. Close your eyes and sit quietly before writing your answers to each question.

### Awareness

1.  Write down the names of some people to whom you characteristically react with a feeling of tension. Then write why you think it is that you have that reaction. In what way would you like the individuals concerned to be different from the way they are?

2.  Choose a specific situation in the recent past that you remember as particularly stressful. What were the elements in that situation that caused you to react with tension and to experience unpleasant emotions? How would you have liked the situation to be different?

3.  Look back at what you wrote in your first answer. Now see if you can write down, for each person, three of his or her good points and three useful things that you have learned about yourself from your interactions with him or her.

4.  Look over what you wrote about the stressful situation. Reflect on it for a moment with your eyes closed. Then write down what you now see, with the perspective of time, that you learned from that situation. Write the main lesson in it for you, and then as many other learnings as you can.

## Acceptance

5.  Review all your answers. Write down what you see about the way in which your attitude (your perspective or point of view) affects your reaction to so-called stressful situations. How much stress is inherent in the situation and how much is caused by your own reaction to the situation, your ongoing point of view?

## Adjustment

6.  How will you handle those kinds of situations the next time they arise? Write down some specific ways in which you can think differently and so reduce the amount of tension you experience in such situations.

7.  Are you feeling self-rejecting or "bad" about what you discovered? That is just another unproductive way of thinking that causes tension, both in you and those around you! What you feel is what you project to others and affects how they, in turn, feel about you. It is important, therefore, to think positively about yourself and to love yourself, not simply for your good qualities, but for your willingness to see your weak areas and work on them.

8.  To help in this positive thinking about yourself, list ten qualities about yourself that you and/or other people appreciate.

9.  Finally, list ten things you are grateful for in your life. (If at the end of every day, you listed ten things or even five that you were grateful for, you would be amazed at the change in your thinking patterns, particularly in the way you feel at the end of a so-called bad day!)

# Self-Discovery Experience

# 5

## How to stop worrying in ten easy stages

### DIRECTIONS:

Sit down quietly in a secluded place where you will not be disturbed. Close your eyes for a few moments, breathe deeply and slowly, and relax. Then begin by selecting a situation about which you are worried.

Worry is another energy drainer. It blocks the flow of prana and sometimes even brings our minds and bodies to a standstill where constructive thought or action seem impossible.

More often than not, worry comes from our vague and often distorted mental projection of the outcome of a situation, rather than from the situation itself. The situation could be one that occurred in the past with effects in the present or future or one in the present or future whose outcome is still undetermined. Worry and the unknown often seem to be companions.

The key to dealing with worry is to demystify it — to set the elements of your worry in front of you for examination, separate the facts from the feared fantasy, and gauge what steps need to be taken for realistic decision-making and action. Action dissolves worry, which is nothing other than indecision or perceived inability to act.

The exercise that follows will assist you in the process of dissecting a worry so you can fearlessly examine its parts. You will find that choosing to take hold of a worry by the simple act of looking at it can be your first step toward relieving yourself of its burden and restoring your view to one of objectivity and optimism.

Oftentimes, once worry has been dispelled, the eye of intuition opens and from within the depths of your prana, your inner energy, an answer emerges that feels very clear and right.

### Awareness

1. On a sheet of paper, briefly describe the situation.
2. How often and how long have you worried about this? When do you worry about it (for example, at mealtimes, bedtime, on your break)?
3. Describe what happens to you, physically and mentally, when you worry about it.
4. What specifically do you imagine might happen? (Elaborate. Write all that you fear might happen.)

## Acceptance

5.  Now what is the worst that could happen?
    a) in the situation?
    b) to you?
6.  Go back and reread all that you've written. Especially examine what you've listed in numbers 4 and 5. Take each point and consider: "Realistically, might this actually occur or is my mind simply fantasizing the worst?"
7.  Now consider, if numbers 4 and 5 did occur, if it is "that bad." Is all really lost?

## Adjustment

8.  Again, consider what you've listed in numbers 4 and 5. Take each point, one at a time, and determine if there are concrete steps you can take now to set the situation in order. For example: "I am worried the roof might cave in." After determining if your concern is realistic (by testing the beams and finding that there is actual evidence), ask: "What concrete steps can I take?" Then list all your choices. In the case of the roof, you could, among other things, move out, call the landlord, or put up new beams.
9.  Where possible, take the concrete steps to remove your worries. Where you see it is not possible, determine simply to drop your worrying and accept what happens. If you can't do anything about the situation, then at least determine to conserve your energy by not worrying. Not only does it not help (you knew that before) but it actually depletes you of physical and mental energy, so that you have less energy to deal with the things that you can do something about.
10. Decide to be in the present, in the moment. Worry is uselessly living in the future. Take care of things the best way you can, and then surrender the rest to life. All the great masters have taught that profound truth. It's what Jesus meant when he spoke of the birds of the air and the lilies of the field, and said "Which of you, by taking thought for the morrow can add one cubit to his stature?" He didn't mean that we should not be practical, or plan ahead; he meant not to waste our energy in continually thinking and worrying about the future!

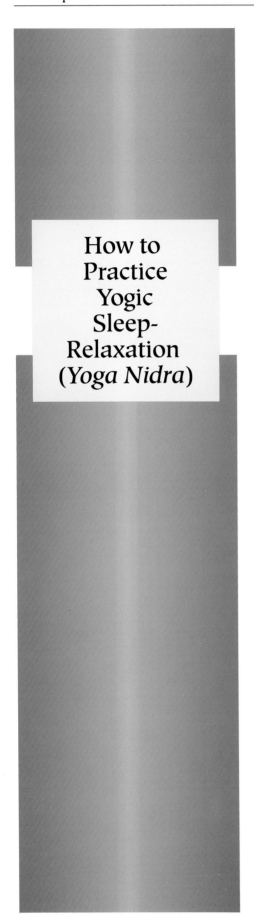

# How to Practice Yogic Sleep-Relaxation (*Yoga Nidra*)

For many centuries yogis have used the technique of yogic sleep-relaxation as a highly effective method of recharging mind and body. You may feel that you are asleep, but in fact this exercise simply takes you to a different level of consciousness that allows the inner intelligence of prana to move freely throughout your system, relaxing, rejuvenating, and healing you on all levels — mental, emotional, and physical.

Follow the instructions below. Try to practice the technique regularly, at least once a day. Soon you'll become old friends with a state that is rightfully yours: the peace and tranquility of a tension-free body and mind. Such an experience will continue to be with you, reflected in what you think, say, and do. The experience will also help your ongoing awareness of your physical and mental states. You will come to recognize your potential for calm awareness, resiliency, and the ability to adjust to unexpected events or demands. Yogic sleep-relaxation may be done any time. By practicing it on a daily basis, you will gradually decrease the level of tension in all of your activities.

Remain in this state for a minimum of fifteen minutes daily. As there is no set maximum time of practice, you may remain in yogic sleep for as long as your schedule permits. At first, you may find it easier to have a close friend quietly read you these instructions, until you have practiced and memorized them. (You may also wish to send for a "KRIPALU by MAIL" catalog and order one of our guided relaxation tapes.)

1.  Prepare your room, your family or co-workers, and yourself. If possible, darken the room and see that the temperature will be comfortable for you. It should be fairly warm, because the body will feel cool due to its slower metabolism, as in sleep. Let your family members or co-workers know that you'd like twenty minutes by yourself. Close the door (perhaps lock it or put up a sign, so you will really feel secure from interruption) and know that this time is just for you. Lie down on your back and close your eyes.

2.  Regulate your breath. Begin to take long, deep, and uniform breaths, gradually slowing down the rate of your breathing. Continue with this breathing throughout each step until you completely lose awareness of it by having sunk deeply into relaxation.

3.  Progressively relax each muscle. As you continue with deep breathing, consciously begin to relax your muscles. Mentally traveling over your body, tell each part to relax, one at a time, from the toes to the top of your head. With each exhalation feel as if you are letting go, breathing out tiredness, stress, tension from that body part. With each inhalation, feel yourself breathing relaxation.

    Relax in this order: your feet, ankles, calves, knees, thighs, hips, abdominal muscles, the muscles of the back, chest, shoulders, arms, and hands. Relax your neck and skull. Then relax your face. Drop any tensions around the eyes and let all facial expression fall away. Relax your forehead, and the sides of your face. Allow your jaw to sag slightly, parting your lips, and relax your tongue.

4.  Relax each organ. Now bring your attention within your body to the internal organs. Without trying to guess their exact location, picture the organs of the abdomen: kidneys, liver, adrenal glands, stomach, intestines, bladder, and reproductive organs.

    As you relax each organ, picture the deep tensions and organic disorders within dissolving at your mental suggestion to relax. Picture your lungs and heart. Feel their pace become slower, more even, free of disturbance or tension. Visualize your brain and imagine that the steady rhythm of breath is cleaning it of all tension — dissolving thoughts and soothing and restoring the millions of cells that lie within it.

5.  Calm your nervous system. When your muscles and organs have become relaxed, consciously begin to relax your nerves. Try to discover where the inner pockets of tension lie within your body. As they reveal themselves to your inner gaze, mentally visualize the incoming breath dissolving these buried tensions. Expel their last vestiges with your exhalation.

    Feel that your tired and overworked nervous channels are closing down, that communication between your brain and nerve centers is being temporarily suspended. Feel that you have completely let go, that your mind is like a clear blue sky with the thoughts as slowly floating clouds. Feel your body growing heavier and heavier as it sinks into the floor.

6.  Calm your mind; let go. Now send your mind as far as it can go from your everyday life. Leave your anxieties and worries, your obligations and responsibilities. Create a strong mental image of a place where you are completely free, completely at peace. Perhaps you will visualize a sunny beach or a silent garden. Retreat into that space, your personal sanctuary, leaving only your body lying on the floor. Be completely in your imagined retreat, in a state devoid of all fears for the future and all regrets over the past. Secure in the knowledge that you are at home, within yourself, allow your conscious mind to drift into a state of blankness, that state in which the inner intelligence of prana works to heal and restore your being thoroughly on all levels.

7.  Come back gently, when you are ready. Stay in this state of sleep-relaxation for as long as you wish. When your consciousness begins to return to your body, do not sit up right away. Instead, linger in the twilight state for a short time, gently stretching your body in the way that feels most natural for you. After a few minutes open your eyes and slowly sit up.

## In Summary:
## Relaxation Is a Way of Life

Relaxation is the result of doing many good things for yourself in your life, little as well as big, from proper diet to a positive attitude in your work. Remember that it comes from bringing about both physical and mental harmony in your life.

After working with the physical approaches to relaxing, you will have keen awareness and energy to enable you to look at the more subtle causes of tension: desires, likes, dislikes, or expectations you may have of yourself or others or that others may have of you. Working on that level of relaxing takes a bit more awareness, honesty, acceptance, and patience. Allow yourself to experience self-esteem through your willingness to look, discover, change, and grow.

Aspire to do good things in your life: (1) accept others through understanding rather than resisting or expecting that they'll change; (2) find one aspect of your work that you like and enjoy it thoroughly, performing it eagerly, and you will begin to gather energy to accept the less inspiring aspects in your work; (3) learn to look upon an unexpected change in events as an opportunity to acquire inner flexibility; (4) take the time to acknowledge the big and small things for which you can feel grateful, starting with a list of five each night, and soon your two hands won't be enough to count all your blessings; and (5) lastly, look upon yourself and others with patience, trust, and love, remembering that we all create our life experiences by our attitudes. Decide that yours will be a more relaxed attitude to life from now on.

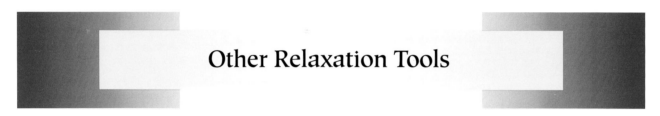

# Other Relaxation Tools

## Biofeedback

Biofeedback has come a long way in the last ten years from an esoteric laboratory research technique to a popular holistic health care tool. The word "biofeedback" simply means feedback from the body, but different machines have been developed to provide that feedback in varying ways. Each machine has essentially the same two functions: to read the body's internal signals and present them to their owner in visual or audible fashion so that he or she can learn to regulate them.

Biofeedback is thus using modern technology to help us do what the sages of the East have been able to do for many centuries, that is, to regulate processes in our bodies that we had regarded as unregulatable: the processes of the so-called involuntary nervous system. Yogis have been able for thousands of years to control their pulse and breathing rate, but for the West that possibility seemed startling and even revolutionary at first.

What are the implications of biofeedback for people interested in holistic health? If you suffer from any form of physical tension, biofeedback is a useful tool for learning how to relax that tension. It is already widely used as a treatment modality for people who suffer from migraine headaches, for instance. By learning to increase the heat in their hands, they draw extra blood there, reducing the congestion in the blood vessels of the brain that seems to be the cause of migraines.

In Kripalu terms, what biofeedback is really doing is reading the subtle signals of prana and relaying them to you. As you become more skilled at reading these signals for yourself and spontaneously bringing relaxation to the different parts of your body, the need for a machine to act as intermediary will be transcended. That, of course, is the ultimate purpose of the Kripalu Approach. We have found, though, that the use of a biofeedback apparatus can be very helpful in starting people on the road to self-regulation and relaxation and in monitoring their progress.

If you have access to biofeedback training in your area, you will find it a rewarding way to begin to get in touch with your prana. To sit and watch a needle on a machine vacillating with every least twitch of your muscles, even with the thoughts that pass through your mind, is fascinating. Try thinking of a situation that makes you really angry and see how the machine responds!

**Note:** There are a number of different kinds of machines on the market to read different manifestations of tension and bodily activity. The most popularly known reads the alpha and other waves of the brain. There are also the Electromyograph which reads muscle tension, primarily in the forehead, and the GSR machines that read galvanic skin response. Some are small and inexpensive enough that you can buy them for home use.

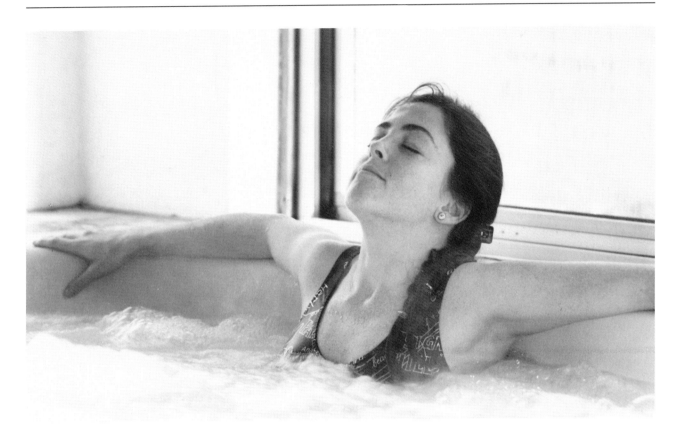

## The Whirlpool

Whirlpools are now so well known that it is probably unnecessary to write about them. We recommend that you try the experience if you have not. If you can't get to ours at Kripalu right away, there's sure to be one available in a health club near you.

The whirlpool is an extremely relaxing and rejuvenating experience. Small, powerful jets of water entering it at different points create turbulence, and standing or sitting against them provides a wonderful gentle massage to the body. The combination of heat and water massage relaxes the muscles and stimulates the whole system so that the bather emerges refreshed and revitalized. It is also great fun since the whirlpool usually accommodates a number of people at once.

An outdoor hot tub has the added exhilaration of enabling you to bathe in steaming water while you take in the fresh outdoors.

## STOP!

How aware are you of your body messages right now? How are you feeling? Is there tension, stiffness, or tiredness in any part of your body? Do you need to get up and stretch? Take some deep breaths? Relax your shoulders? Rest your eyes? Rest your mind? Close your eyes for a minute and take some long, slow, deep breaths to enable you to get in touch with your experience. Then respond to what your body is asking you to do.

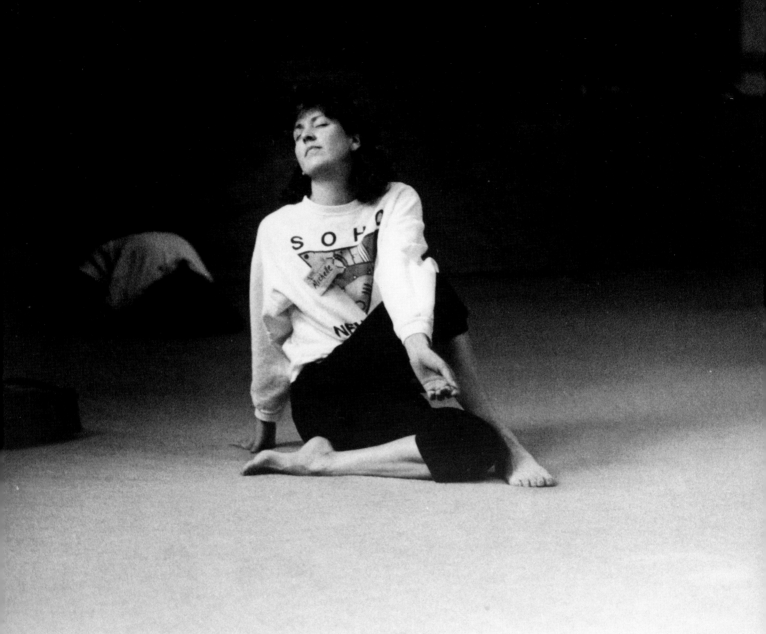

# *The Second Pathway*

getting to know and love your body

# Befriending Your Body

*"The body is the only vehicle that we have on this earth
to experience life and to reach our highest potential."*

Yogi Amrit Desai

Where does health begin? Most of us would say "with the body." Yet if we look at our lives objectively and honestly, we may see that we don't honor our bodies as much as our belief in their importance would warrant. Instead, we expect them to function smoothly and give us no trouble, like a brand new car, and we are surprised and even angry when they break down.

The signals of the body that can help us eliminate sickness and disease from our lives are there for us to hear, however, if we listen. If we learn to love and care for our bodies, they will more than repay us by the quality of life they allow us to experience. So we need to befriend our bodies; to respect them and reacquaint ourselves with how they function, why they malfunction, what their needs are, and how to provide for those needs.

The Kripalu Approach teaches us to begin with the body. This chapter will show you a number of ways to become reacquainted with your body and learn to treat it more lovingly. Whatever your present state of health and mobility, you can improve it if you know how, and that will enrich your whole experience of life. What counts is not how mobile or disease-free you are, but how sensitive and caring you are to recognizing and meeting the needs of your body.

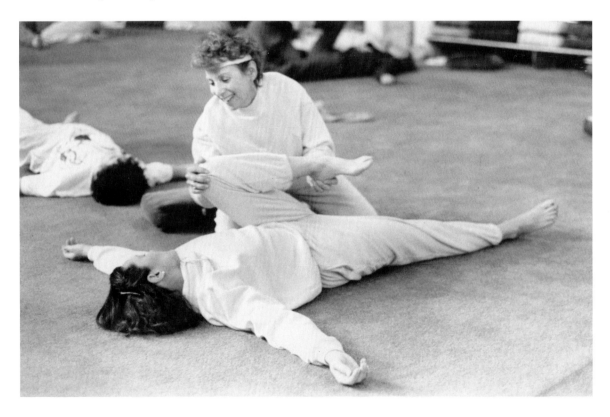

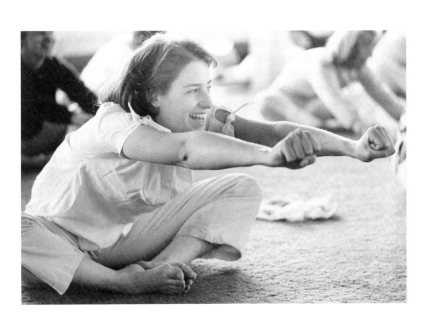

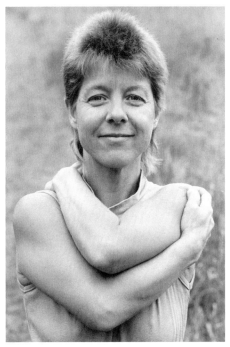

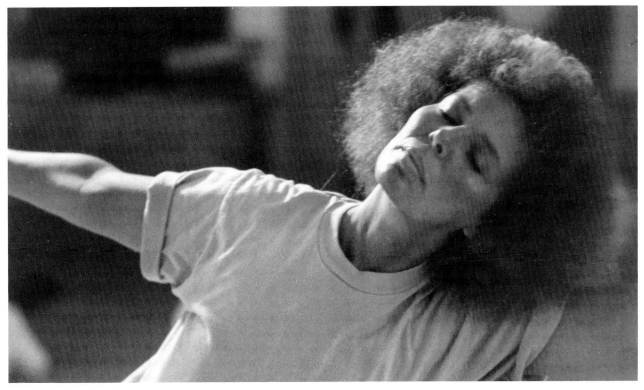

# Self-Discovery Experience

# 6

## How well do you know your body?

### DIRECTIONS:

Sit in a comfortable position with your eyes closed and enter into relaxation by breathing deeply and regularly and allowing your mind to become quiet. Then read the following questions and reflect on each one, again with your eyes closed. Allow the questions to be an experience rather than a thinking process.

### Awareness

1. How does your body feel to you as a rule? Healthy? Fit? Energetic? Sluggish? Supple? Jot down a few words to describe it.

2. Go through your whole body mentally, stopping at each part (head, face, neck, hands, etc.) and try to feel and visualize it clearly. Notice whether there is any tension or tiredness, any aches or pains, that you were not aware of before you stopped to check it out.

3. Now try to visualize the inner organs of your digestive and circulatory systems and your breathing mechanism, one after the other. See if you can become more aware of how they are functioning right now. Feel any blockages or pockets of tension or irregularities.

## Acceptance

Ask yourself:

4. Am I aware of what is happening in my body, or do I tend to take it for granted?

5. Am I so busy doing what I'm doing and thinking of other things, that I hardly ever pay attention to how my body is functioning?

6. Does my body send messages to me that I may not always hear because of the noise in my mind?

## Adjustment

Now that you have become more attuned to your body, it makes sense to think of ways you can continue to be conscious of what is happening inside it.

Ask yourself:

7. What can I do to become more aware of the functioning of my body? (For example, "I can stop from time to time throughout the day and check in" or "I can take more time for relaxation.")

8. What did I notice just now about my body that I particularly need to pay more attention to? (For example, "I noticed pain and stiffness in my neck" or "There seem to be digestive problems I was not aware of.")

9. Write down specific ways in which you can make changes that will help you become more attuned to your body and its needs.

# Yoga and Holistic Health

In the West, yoga is generally known as a system of physical exercise that is used to help slim the body and make it more flexible and youthful and to calm the mind and free it of tension and worry. But that is merely one branch of yoga known as Hatha Yoga.

Yoga is, in fact, a complete science that has many branches. It is one of the most ancient and complete systems of self-development and holistic health that the world has known. Both Hatha Yoga postures and the philosophical realizations that go with them emerged spontaneously from deep meditation experiences of ascetics of ancient India at least 6,000 years ago.

Yoga (which means "union" or "wholeness"), though subsequently developed into a precise science, is also a great art. It is scientific because it consists of specific, time-tested techniques with precise and predictable results, and it is an art because it is ultimately a highly personal experience and form of self-expression.

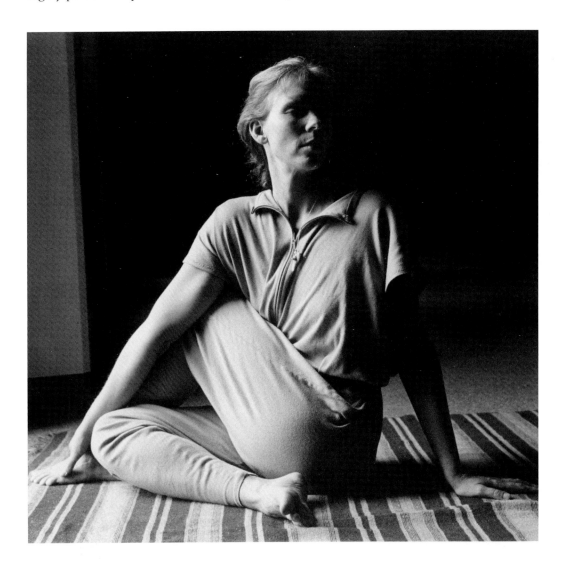

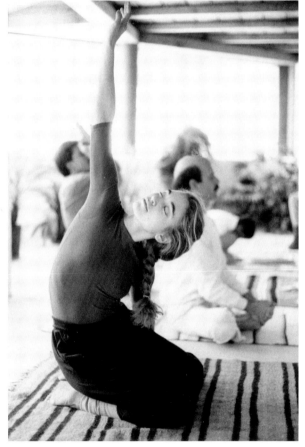

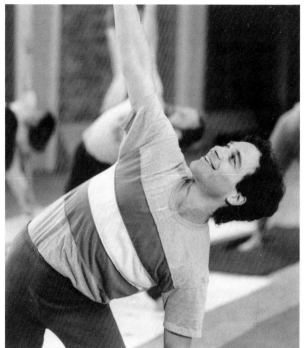

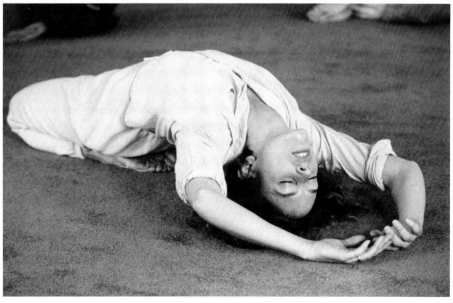

## Hatha Yoga — The Gentle Exercise System for All Ages, Shapes, and Sizes

Hatha Yoga postures (known as asanas) are very different from other forms of physical exercise. They are designed not so much for muscle development as to bring about the balanced functioning of the nerves and glands. These methods are safe and simple and can be easily grasped and mastered with consistent practice by almost anyone.

Because yoga exercises are done slowly, they do not require a great deal of stamina and can consequently be practiced and enjoyed by young and old. Those with a physical disease or disability can also benefit from doing yoga; it has even been successfully taught to people who are bedridden and those in wheelchairs! The postures, when done properly, never strain the body but serve to enhance and stimulate the functioning of the inner organs.

Although Hatha Yoga does work on external physical and emotional problems, its main focus is on the root causes of these problems, which are usually found in the functioning of the nerves and glands or in the mind. Obesity, for example, is not necessarily caused by overeating alone. It can be the result of a malfunctioning thyroid gland, of agitated and tense nerves, or of outdated thinking patterns.

Yoga postures work directly on relaxing deep tensions. At the same time, they affect the functioning of the glandular and nervous systems, adding strength, resilience, and harmony. As a result, the postures bring about a deep and lasting change in our state of health by focusing on the very source of our physical problems.

The glandular and nervous systems of the body are the main systems responsible for controlling our thought patterns, emotional reactions, and degree of

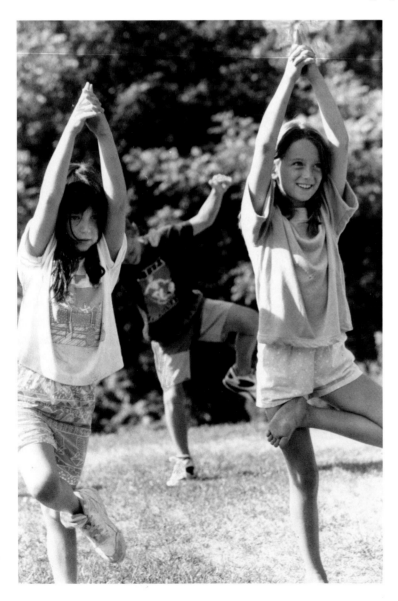

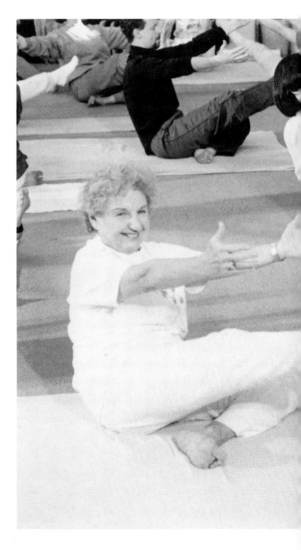

happiness or unhappiness. All physical and mental processes are regulated by the glands and nerves — if they are not functioning properly, we may be medically alive, but we are not alive in the true sense of being holistically healthy. Even achieving a state of physical health will not in itself satisfy our deeper inner needs. So Hatha Yoga is not an end in itself but a means, a stepping stone, to higher levels of consciousness. The ultimate purpose of yoga is to unite the forces of *Ha* (positive, masculine energy symbolized by the sun) and *Tha* (negative, feminine energy symbolized by the moon).

These complementary energies exist within each of us and give rise to our experience of polarity and the conflict of duality as we live in the world. When the energies of *Ha* and *Tha* are united within us through the practice of yoga, it is possible for us to transcend these apparent conflicts and experience the essential unity of all life.

## TYPES OF YOGA

Most people begin their yoga practice with Hatha Yoga, but there are other forms of yoga that lead toward the goal of integration of body, mind, and spirit. The other forms of yoga practice are described in the first written compilation of yogic knowledge, Pantanjali's *Yoga Sutras*, which was composed about 200 B.C. They are outlined below:

*Karma Yoga:* wholeness through service, work, and action.

*Jnana Yoga:* wholeness through knowledge and study.

*Bhakti Yoga:* wholeness through devotion and selfless love.

*Mantra Yoga:* wholeness through sound, vibration, and speech.

*Raja Yoga:* wholeness through control of the mind.

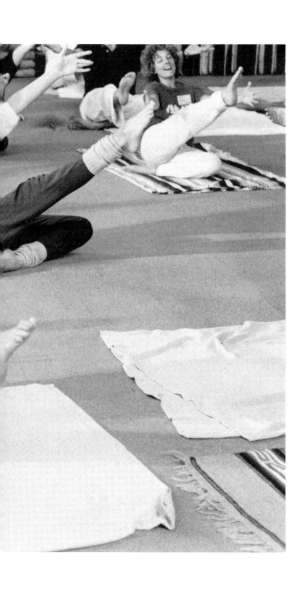

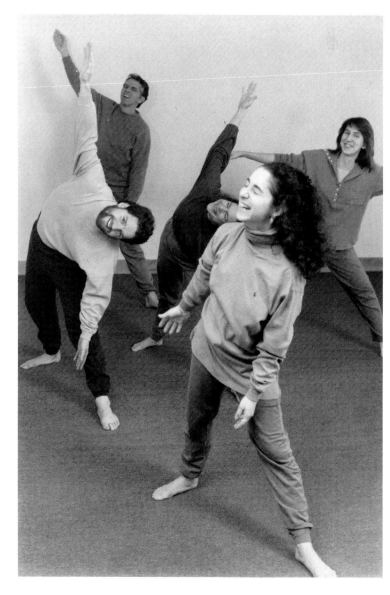

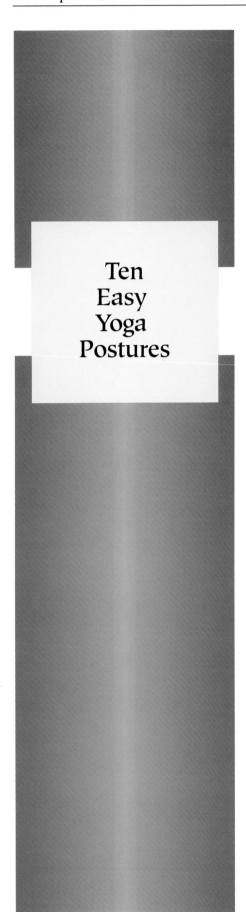

# Ten Easy Yoga Postures

Like any other form of exercise, yoga postures are best practiced after some limbering up has taken place to warm up the body and loosen the muscles. The first series of movements suggested here are for that purpose. Called "The Wake-up Routine" because they are a wonderful way to wake up in the early morning, these simple movements are also an excellent way to start your yoga practice.

As with all yoga postures, carry the movements out slowly and gently, without any strain. You should make a moderate effort to stretch your body a little more than usual, but never to the point of extreme discomfort or pain. The purpose is to experience your body and its capabilities and to enjoy the pleasant feeling of stretching, like a cat or a small child.

Remember that you are not competing with anyone, not even yourself. You do not need to perform the postures perfectly, but simply to feel your body in new ways or with a new awareness and learn from what it is telling you. As much as possible, do these postures with your eyes closed, as this will heighten your sense of contact with your body and your level of relaxation.

**NOTE:** The postures have been presented in a specific order so that each bend in one direction is followed by a complementary bend in the opposite direction. It is always advisable to do postures in complementary pairs, because it maintains the balance of the body.

## Why We Limber Up in the Morning

Waking up in the morning is like the birth of a baby: it can thrust you into the world abruptly, even jarringly, or it can be a gentle, loving entry into the daylight that will keep you calm, serene, and centered all day long. The key is to move slowly, allowing your body time to make the delicate transition from the sleeping, passive mode to the alert, active state.

Muscles and joints that have stiffened during the night's inactivity must be gently stretched and mobilized, particularly the spine. The body's energy needs to be stimulated gently. The lungs need to be opened so that you again inhale deeply and fully after a night of shallow breathing when the body required less oxygen.

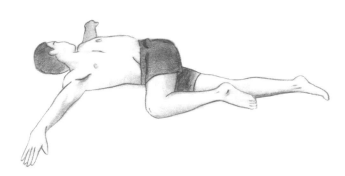

## The Wake-up Routine

1. Remain in bed (if your bed is not too soft) or gently rise and lie on the floor beside the bed. Lie on your back with legs straight and arms comfortably at your sides. Relax.

2. Clasp your hands on your stomach, interlacing the fingers. Invert your palms and stretch them downward toward your feet, straightening your arms. Now slowly (all movements should be very slow unless otherwise indicated) begin to lift your arms into the air, breathing in deeply and slowly, and bring your arms down to the floor or bed behind/above your head, fully stretching out. Exhaling, stretch and arch your back, loosening up your spine.

3. On the next exhalation, unclasp your hands and, as you inhale, stretch the right arm and leg in a straight line, making that side of your body longer than the other and lifting your right hip slightly. Exhale and relax. Now repeat with your left arm and leg. Inhale deeply and stretch fully, lifting your left hip. Relax.

4. Lift your arms again until your hands are directly above your shoulders (toward the ceiling). Release your hands and gently rotate them around the wrists, several times in each direction, making complete circles

5. You may need to be on the floor for this next exercise in order to have enough room for your arms: Gently lower your arms to the sides until they rest on the bed or floor and are directly out from your shoulders.

Inhaling, slowly raise your right knee, sliding the right foot along the ground until it is next to your left knee. Exhaling, slowly twist your body, bringing your right knee over toward the ground on the outside of your left thigh and turning your head to the right.

Don't strain in this posture. Be very relaxed and enjoy the stretch. Breathe deeply. Now, exhaling slowly, return to center and slide your foot back to its starting position beside the other foot. Relax for a moment, breathing deeply. Then, inhaling, repeat the twist on the other side. Relax.

6. Again, being on the floor will be helpful to provide enough space around you. Gently come to a seated position with your knees up to your chest, feet on the floor, hands clasped under your knees, back rounded, and head bent forward. Gently begin to roll back onto your upper back, keeping the spine well curved and the head tucked in (this is important). Rock backward and forward like this about a dozen times, fairly briskly, so that the momentum going back will help you come forward. Straighten your legs as you rock back; bend them again as you return. Breathe in as you rock back, out as you rock forward. Then relax on your back.

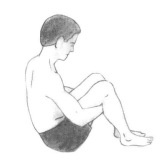

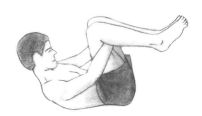

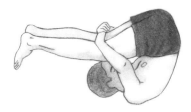

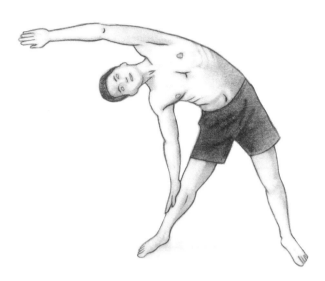

## 1.   The Triangle (*Trikonasana*)

**BENEFITS:**
1.   Provides alternate flexing and relaxing of the trunk's lateral and dorsal muscles, promoting resilience in the spine and proper placement in the bones and muscles of the hips.
2.   Invigorates the abdominal muscles and organs.
3.   Tones the hamstring muscles and strengthens the sciatic nerves.

**INSTRUCTIONS:**

**Triangle 1:**
1.   Stand with your legs about shoulder width apart, feet turned slightly outward. Exhale.
2.   Inhale as you raise both arms out to your sides until they are in line with your shoulders, with palms facing down.
3.   Exhale as you bend from your waist to the right, pressing your left hip slightly to the left. Stretch your left arm over your head, parallel to the floor and close to your ear. Allow your right hand to glide along your thigh toward your ankle, as far as is comfortable. Keep your legs straight and your pelvis forward. Do not twist at the waist, shoulders, or legs.
4.   Inhaling, slowly raise your body to the original position.
5.   Repeat on the opposite side, bending sideways to the left.
6.   Inhale as you return to the standing position.
7.   Exhale as you lower your arms and bring your feet together. Relax.

**Triangle 2:**
1.   Stand as in Triangle 1. Exhale.
2.   As you inhale, raise your arms sideways to shoulder level with your palms facing down.
3.   As you exhale, twist your upper body to the right, then bend at the waist, keeping your arms in a straight line, so that your right arm rotates up with fingers reaching toward the ceiling as you lower your left hand to the outside of your right foot. Turn your head and look at your right thumb. Keep your legs straight. Hold to comfort level.
4.   Inhale as you return to standing and bring your arms in line with your shoulders.
5.   Exhale as you turn your upper body to face the front.
6.   Repeat in the opposite direction.
7.   Exhale as you lower your arms and bring your feet together. Relax.

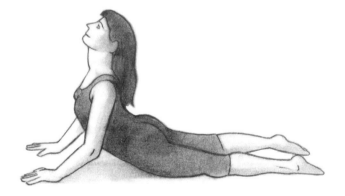

## 2.   The Cobra (*Bhujangasana*)

**BENEFITS:**
1.   Helps to regulate the functions of the gonads and uterus and to prevent and relieve menstrual disorders.
2.   Stimulates and relaxes vertebrae from the neck to the base of the spine. Strengthens and tones weak spinal muscles.
3.   Recharges the entire abdominal region with an abundant flow of blood. Rejuvenates the kidneys. Stimulates the thyroid and adrenal glands. Trims abdominal fat and tones the buttocks.
4.   Helps to relieve the tension of backache caused by long hours of sitting, walking, or driving. An excellent posture to do before going to sleep at night.

## HINTS AND CAUTIONS:

As with all yoga postures, sudden or jerking movements may cause stiffness. Train your body gently through consistent practice rather than by forcing or fighting it. You should rise up to the Cobra position using only the muscles of your back and not your arms. You may want to place your palms on the back of your thighs and rise up with no support. The Cobra should not be done after the third month of pregnancy.

## INSTRUCTIONS:

1. Lie on your abdomen and relax completely. Place your forehead on the floor and your palms down, with fingertips in line with your shoulders. Keep your elbows off the floor and your legs together with toes pointed. Exhale deeply.

2. Inhaling, slowly and gracefully raise your forehead, nose, and chin, followed by your shoulders and chest, in one continuous movement. Use your arms to maintain your balance, but not for support. Keep your elbows bent and your shoulders down.

3. Arch your head back and look up. Your navel and hips remain on the floor. Hold the position, remaining relaxed.

4. Exhaling, slowly uncurl your spine and lower your chest, chin, nose, and then your eyes until your forehead rests again on the floor.

5. Repeat the Cobra two or three times.

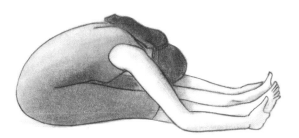

# 3.  The Head-to-Knee Posture
## (Paschimottanasana)

## BENEFITS:

1. Stretches and strengthens the nerves of the lower back, thereby helping to prevent functional disorders of the stomach, liver, spleen, kidneys, and intestines.

2. Improves appetite and stimulates underactive liver and kidneys. Helps to relieve constipation and indigestion.

3. Streamlines the abdomen. Slims and tones hips and thighs.

4. Helps prevent hemorrhoids.

5. Provides a powerful stretch for the entire back from the neck to the heels.

6. Develops and tones the back and the hamstring muscles of the legs.

7. Promotes elasticity of the spine and strengthens the vital nerve plexuses of the spine. Stretches and strengthens the crucial sciatic nerve.

## HINTS AND CAUTIONS:

Avoid sudden movement and strain, as in every yoga posture. Do not force your head to touch your knees if this is very uncomfortable or painful. Simply come as close as you can without strain and you will still gain all the benefits. Concentrate on bending from the lower back rather than from the shoulders and upper back. Your knees should be straight in order to derive full benefit from this posture. If you suffer from any back injury or from severe constipation, practice this posture cautiously, increasing the holding time very gradually.

## INSTRUCTIONS:

1. Sit on the floor with both legs stretched out in front of you and your back straight. Exhale deeply.

2. Inhaling, slowly raise your arms above your head without bending your elbows. Stretch upwards from the waist.

3. Exhaling, bend from the hips, stretching forward over your knees. Bring your head as close as you comfortably can to your knees. Hold onto your feet, ankles, calves, or wherever you can reach comfortably without straining. Breathe deeply.

4. Inhaling, slowly sit up again, stretching your arms above your head.

5. Exhaling, lower your arms gracefully. Relax, breathing deeply.

An easier, beginner's version is to bend one leg, placing the sole of your foot against the inside of the opposite leg, as high on the leg as possible. Then bend forward over your outstretched leg, following the same steps listed for the Head-to-Knee posture. Be sure that the straightened leg remains flat on the floor and straight out from the hip (not slanted). Repeat on the other side.

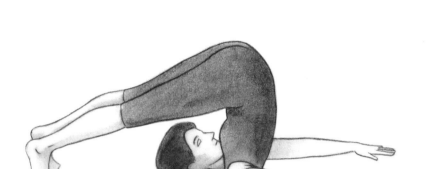

## 4.   The Plough (*Halasana*)

**BENEFITS:**

1. Aligns the vertebrae and brings a fresh supply of blood to the nerve centers along the spine. An ideal orthopedic exercise, helping to correct spinal irregularities in children and minor dislocations of the vertebrae in adults.
2. Enhances body symmetry and strengthens the back muscles.
3. Rejuvenates and cleanses the gonads, pancreas, liver, spleen, kidneys, and adrenal glands.
4. Helps regulate the function of the thyroid, calming the nerves and blessing the entire system with youthfulness.
5. Helps relieve exhaustion, fatigue, and stiffness of the back and shoulders.
6. Diminishes facial lines and wrinkles.
7. Trims away accumulated fat in the abdomen and hips. Tones and firms the legs.
8. Strengthens the organs of the neck and thorax.
9. Stimulates brain activity, relieving headaches and disorders caused by anemia of the brain. Increases blood circulation to the brain and clears the mind.

**HINTS AND CAUTIONS:**

Again, be careful not to strain by overly vigorous movements. Do not attempt to force your toes to the floor; it is not necessary. If the Plough is difficult for you, try this preparation: Lie on the floor with the top of your head about one-and-a-half feet from a wall. As your feet come over your head into the Plough, brace them against the wall, then simply walk down the wall to the floor. You can also rock into the Plough position.

**INSTRUCTIONS:**

1. Lying on your back, place your arms close to your sides, palms down. Keep both knees straight. Exhale.
2. Inhaling, press your palms against the floor and slowly raise your legs until they point to the ceiling.
3. Exhaling, lower your legs over your head until your feet touch the floor behind your head or come as close as is comfortable. Do not bend your knees.
4. Hold that position, supporting your hips with your hands if necessary to maintain balance. Breathe deeply and slowly.
5. Inhaling, slowly lower your back, vertebra by vertebra, until your hips have reached the floor and your legs are toward the ceiling once more. Exhaling, slowly lower your legs to the floor without bending your knees. (Beginners: Bend your knees toward your forehead and press your hands into the ground until your lower back is on the floor. Then straighten your legs again and lower them slowly.)

Relax and breathe normally, experiencing the benefits.

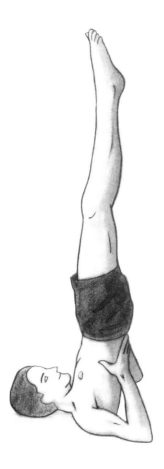

7.  Eases constipation and indigestion.
8.  Nourishes facial skin, scalp, and hair roots, helping to erase wrinkles, and improving general complexion.
9.  Regulates the thymus gland, which controls physical and mental development. Highly recommended for growing children and adolescents.
10. **NOTE:** The Reverse Posture, given as a preparation for the Shoulderstand, primarily benefits the gonads and sends increased circulation to the face.

## HINTS AND CAUTIONS:

The Shoulderstand is a most precious gift, given to humanity by the ancient yogis. Its Sanskrit name means "the exercise that benefits the entire body." It produces many of the rejuvenation effects of the more difficult inverted postures. Persons suffering from extremely high or low blood pressure, organic thyroid disorders, chronic nasal catarrh, glaucoma, detached retina, or weak eye capillaries should consult their physician before attempting the Shoulderstand.

## INSTRUCTIONS:

First, an easy version: The Reverse Posture.

1.  Lie on your back with your hands at your sides, palms facing down, with your feet together and legs straight. Exhale deeply.
2.  Inhaling, slowly raise your straightened legs toward the ceiling.
3.  Exhaling, lift your hips and lower your legs toward the floor over your head. Inhaling, lift your legs to a sixty-degree angle with the floor, supporting your hips with your hands. Hold the position and breathe deeply.
4.  Exhaling, lower your legs toward the floor over your head. Then, inhaling, slowly and steadily lower your back to the floor. Exhaling again, return your legs to the floor. Relax.

(Beginners: To come out of the posture, bend your knees toward your forehead and press your hands into the ground to lower your trunk slowly. When your lower back is on the floor, stretch your legs out and gently and slowly lower them to the floor.)

The Shoulderstand (after one week of practice of the Reverse Posture).

1.  Lie on your back, as for the Reverse Posture. Press down on the floor with your palms. Inhaling, gradually raise your straightened legs to a perpendicular position, keeping your knees straight.
2.  Exhaling, slowly raise your hips and lower your legs over your head. Support your upper back with your hands, bringing your entire body into a vertical position as you inhale. Point your toes toward the ceiling. Make your body as straight as possible.
3.  While holding this position, keep your chin firmly pressed against your breastbone. Breathe deeply.
4.  Exhaling, lower your legs over your head. Inhaling, lower your back to the floor, reversing your upward movement. Finally, exhaling, bring your legs back to the floor. Do not repeat immediately. Relax and breathe deeply.

## 5.   The Shoulderstand (*Sarvangasana*)

## BENEFITS:

1.  Helps to regulate both over- and underweight by normalizing the functions of the thyroid and parathyroid glands through the pressure of the chin. These glands regulate metabolic processes, heartbeat, and blood pressure. Every vital organ is affected by the well-being of the thyroid gland.
2.  Sends a generous supply of blood to the organs in the upper portion of the body, helping to prevent and relieve such ailments as throat and chest colds, sore throats, bronchitis, asthma, and headaches. The heart is relieved for a time of the strain of pumping blood against gravity to the demanding organs of the head and neck.
3.  Improves circulation, relieving pressure on the blood vessels and making them resilient. Helps prevent and relieve varicose veins and hemorrhoids.
4.  Helps to correct displacement of vital internal glands and organs, especially the female organs. Benefits those suffering from female disorders.
5.  Tones the gonads and helps maintain the vitality of the entire body. Restores dissipated energy, bringing new youth to the entire system.
6.  Effectively combats insomnia and nervous disorders, as well as sluggishness and indolence, by regulating glandular functions.

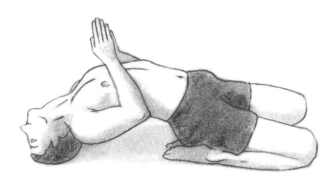

# 6.    The Fish (*Matsyasana*)

**BENEFITS:**

1.    Helps to correct lung displacement in the thoracic cavity caused by restricted and long immobilization (such as sitting at a desk), thus increasing lung capacity. Helps prevent and relieve asthma.

2.    Eases curved and stiffened backs.

3.    Flushes muscles of the spine, as well as the abdominal and neck organs. Excellent for colds and swollen tonsils.

4.    Increases circulation to the back and stimulates the nerves of the spinal cord, sympathetic nervous system and the solar plexus.

5.    Tones the abdominal viscera (the liver, spleen, and pelvic organs).

6.    Helps alleviate painful hemorrhoids.

7.    Benefits the adrenal glands, gonads, and pancreas.

8.    Tones the chest and back, improving posture and thus affecting psychological attitudes.

**HINTS AND CAUTIONS:**

The Fish is often done immediately following the Shoulderstand, as it both complements and stabilizes the stretch given to the neck muscles by the Shoulderstand.

**INSTRUCTIONS:**

1.    Lie on your back with your legs tucked underneath your buttocks, and your arms resting at your sides. Relax, and exhale deeply.

2.    Inhaling, use your elbows for support and arch your back between your hips and the top of your head. Rest the top of your head on the floor. (Beginners may find it easier to place the hands palms down under the hips and arch up with the support of the elbows.)

3.    Hold the posture. Breathe deeply. If you feel secure, lift your elbows and join your hands over your chest in prayer position.

4.    Exhaling, bring your arms out of prayer position and place your elbows once again on the floor for support. Then gently lower your head and then your back, supporting your body with your elbows. Release your hands and relax. Do not repeat the Fish a second time.

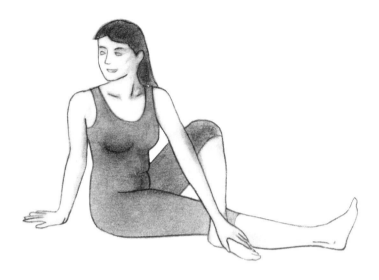

## 7.   The Twist (*Ardha Matsyendrasana*)

**BENEFITS:**

1. Helps prevent lumbago, backstrain, and certain forms of sciatica.
2. Tones sluggish kidneys and adrenals, aiding in the process of diuresis.
3. Decongests a clogged liver and spleen. Combats obesity, constipation, and indigestion by increasing the peristaltic movement of the bowels.
4. Helps relieve asthma.
5. Removes calcium deposits of the shoulders, freeing shoulder movement. Helps overcome stiffness of the neck.
6. Strengthens and elasticizes the spine: helps correct stooped shoulders, bent back, defective posture, and minor spinal deformities.

**INSTRUCTIONS:**

### Version One (an easy version):
### The Half Twist

1. Sit on the floor with your legs stretched in front of you. Bend your right leg, placing the sole of your right foot on the floor to the left of your left knee.
2. Place your left palm on the floor behind your back on the left side. Point your fingers away from your body. Keep your back very straight and your arm as close as possible to your back.
3. Place your right arm along the inside of your right leg. Grasp your right ankle. Exhale deeply.
4. Sitting erect and inhaling, turn slowly to the left until

you are looking at the wall behind you. Hold the position, breathing deeply. Do not change the upright position of your right knee.

5. Exhaling, release the posture slowly. Relax.
6. Repeat in the opposite direction.
7. Repeat for a total of two or three times on each side.

### Version Two: The Full Twist
### (after three to four weeks of practice of the Half Twist)

1. Sit on your heels.
2. Shift your hips so that you are sitting on the floor, to the left of both feet.
3. Grasp your right ankle with the right hand and place it on the outside of your left knee. Keep your back straight and your knee upright.
4. Raise your arms so that they are perpendicular to your body.
5. Inhaling, twist to the right, bringing your left arm to the right (outside) of your right knee and clasping the right ankle or foot with your left hand. Place the right hand on the floor behind and very close to your back, with your fingers pointing away from your body.
6. Now look over your right shoulder, twisting from the base of your spine up to your neck. Hold this position. Placing gentle pressure on your right (raised) leg with your left elbow will increase the twist.
7. Exhaling, slowly return to the starting position. Release the position and relax.
8. Repeat in the opposite direction.

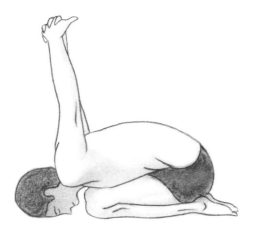

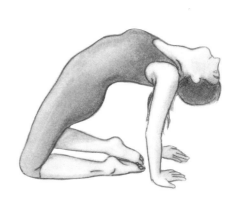

## 8.   *Yoga Mudra*

**BENEFITS**:
1.  Expands the lungs and stimulates the lung cells.
2.  Stimulates the peristaltic movement of the bowels, helping to relieve constipation.
3.  Strengthens the nerves and muscles of the abdominal and pelvic areas.
4.  Recharges the colon and intestinal nerve, aligning the abdominal organs by an external and internal massage.
5.  Develops the chest, and exercises seldom used arm and shoulder muscles.
6.  Provides relief from tension throughout the trunk area caused by extended periods of sitting and bending.
7.  Improves general posture, thus increasing self-confidence.

**HINTS AND CAUTIONS:**
If you suffer from chronic constipation, practice this posture gently, releasing it slowly and avoiding jerky movements.

**INSTRUCTIONS:**
1.  Assume a kneeling position, placing your palms on your knees. Exhale deeply.
2.  Inhaling, bring your arms behind your back in a slow and steady circular motion. Interlock your fingers and straighten your arms. Do not change the position of your palms.
3.  Exhaling, bend forward, raising your arms as high as possible, until your forehead touches the floor.
4.  Hold the position. For an additional stretch you may bring your chin to the floor.
5.  Inhaling, sit up slowly. Exhaling, let your arms return to your knees on their own accord. (The spontaneous movement you may experience at this stage is a preliminary experience of prana-directed movement.)
6.  Repeat the posture a second time.

## 9.   **The Camel** (*Ushtrasana*)

**BENEFITS:**
1.  Eases back tension and increases spinal flexibility. Helps to correct a curved back and rounded shoulders.
2.  Develops the chest and firms the muscles of the upper arms, thighs, and abdomen.
3.  Strengthens and elasticizes the feet.
4.  Gently massages the heart.
5.  Rejuvenates the thyroid and gonads, bestowing youthfulness on your entire system.

**HINTS AND CAUTIONS:**
As back stretching is difficult for many people, proceed slowly. Avoid tensing your muscles as this will inhibit both flexibility and gradual, graceful movement. If you are suffering from a hernia, do not practice the Camel.

**INSTRUCTIONS:**
1.  Assume a kneeling position. Place your palms on your knees. Exhale deeply.
2.  Inhaling, slowly bring your arms behind your back. Place your palms on the floor, directly behind your feet. Point your fingers away from your body.
3.  Exhaling, shift your weight to your arms, dropping your head back.
4.  Inhaling, raise your hips and arch your back. Shift your body weight onto your knees and thighs.
5.  Hold the posture to comfort level. Breathe deeply.
6.  Exhaling, lower your hips to your heels. Keep your hands on the floor and your head back.
7.  Inhaling, raise your head and shoulders.
8.  Exhaling, slowly bring your hands onto your knees. Relax.

Repeat two or three times.

## 10.   The Sun Salutation (*Surya Namaskar*)

**BENEFITS:**

1. Tones the digestive system by alternately stretching and compressing the abdominal region. Massages the liver, stomach, spleen, intestines, and kidneys. Stimulates the digestive process and helps to relieve constipation and dyspepsia.

2. Thoroughly ventilates the lungs. Oxygenates the blood and removes carbon dioxide and other toxic gases from the respiratory tract.

3. Increases circulation throughout the entire system. Brings warmth, vigor, and vitality to the limbs of the body.

4. Stretches and massages the spinal column, toning and regulating functions of the sympathetic and parasympathetic nervous systems. Helps dispel insomnia, hypertension, worry, and anxiety. Improves the memory.

5. Helps normalize the functions of the endocrine glands, relieving emotional stress and tension. The thyroid gland is especially benefited by the Sun Salutation.

6. Refreshes and tones the skin, helping to remove premature wrinkles and prevent sagging.

7. Strengthens and tones all the muscles of the body, especially those in the back. Helps relieve and prevent backaches caused by long hours of standing or sitting.

8. Tones and firms the upper arms, bust, and shoulders. Helps to correct posture and bestow a sense of balance, grace, and self-confidence.

9. Affects activity in the uterus and ovaries, helping to regulate the menstrual cycle. Relieves and prevents menstrual discomfort. Facilitates easy childbirth.

10. Tones and slims the waist, thighs, hips, and buttocks. Helps remove excess weight from any area of the body that may be improperly proportioned as a result of overeating or lack of exercise.

11. Helps to prevent the loss of hair and slows the graying process.

12. Affects each cell of the body, bestowing an overall feeling of well-being, vitality, and peace. As a result, the mind is able to function with greater clarity and calmness.

**HINTS AND CAUTIONS:**

This exercise is traditionally practiced in the early morning as a salute to the sun, nature's symbol of health and long life. It is a combination of asanas and breathing exercises that, when mastered, produces a meditative flow of bodily movement. The Sun Salutation may be used as a warm-up before your daily yoga exercises, as it limbers the spine as well as all the muscles of the body and invigorates the entire system.

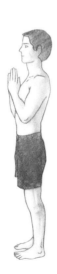

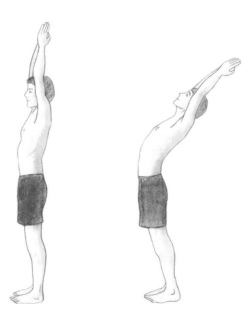

1. Stand erect with your feet and legs together. Join your palms in prayer position in front of your chest, with your elbows pointed downward. Interlock your thumbs.

2. Without releasing your hands, slowly raise your arms over your head as you inhale. Keeping your head between your arms, bend slightly backward with breath held. Keep your knees locked and your feet firmly positioned on the floor.

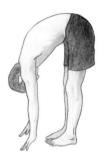

3.   Exhaling, bend forward from the hips, placing your hands palms down on the floor on either side of your feet, with your toes and fingertips in a straight line. If this is too difficult, bend your knees slightly.

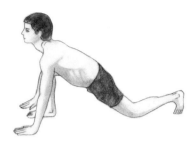

4.   Inhaling, stretch your right leg behind you as far as possible. Rest your right knee on the floor and curl your toes under your foot. Your left foot should remain stationary between your hands, with your chest touching your left thigh and knee. Look up and arch your back, stretching your head, neck, and chest.

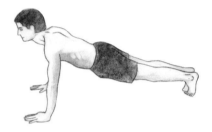

5.   Hold your breath as you straighten your right knee and bring your left leg back to join it. Both feet and legs should be together. Straighten your arms with your palms still on the floor so that your entire body forms a straight line (the push-up position).

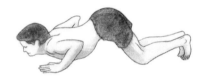

6.   Exhaling, gradually lower your body, touching your knees, chest, and forehead to the floor. If it is difficult to place the forehead on the floor, you can touch the chin instead. The buttocks remain raised.

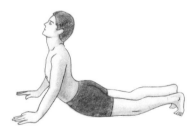

7.   Inhale and lower your hips and abdomen to the floor, uncurling your toes and relaxing your head, neck, and chest. Arching your back as in the Cobra, straighten your arms and rest your weight on your hands. The hips and thighs should remain on the floor.

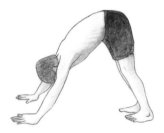

8.   Curl your toes under your feet once again. Exhaling, lift your hips, resting your weight on your hands and feet. Your body should form a triangle, with your head between your arms. Keep your feet flat on the floor by pressing your heels down. If this is difficult, walk toward the hands until your feet are flat. Press your torso toward your legs, so that your spine curves inward.

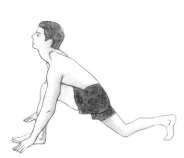

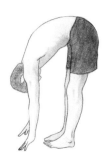

9.  Inhaling, take a long and quick step forward and place your right foot between your hands. Keep your left leg stretched behind you and lower your left knee to the floor. Then raise your head and arch your back. (This position is the reverse of step number 4.)

10.  Exhaling, bring your left leg forward and place it next to your right leg. Straighten your knees. Place your palms flat on the floor on either side of your feet. Bring your head toward your knees.

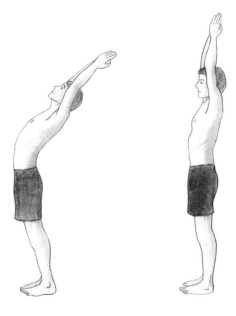

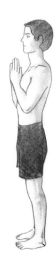

11.  Inhale and slowly straighten up, stretching your arms and arching back as in step number 2.

12.  Exhaling, gradually lower your arms back into prayer position. Stand still with your eyes closed for a few seconds.

# Yogic Breathing and Prana

### Life and Breath

Breathing is the most basic function of human life, for what we call life begins with our first breath in and ends with our last breath out. Life is the process contained between these two breaths and sustained by the intervening breaths. Breath, then, is life, for although we can survive for many days without food and water, we can survive for only a few minutes without breathing.

Because the relationship between breath and life is so intimate, our way of breathing has a profound effect on the quality of our lives. Yet how many of us are aware of our manner of breathing at any given moment? Or of how it is affecting our body, mind, and emotions? The act of breathing, for most of us, is an automatic process that we take completely for granted until a problem develops.

What we call normal breathing is usually a shallow, superficial process involving just the upper portion of the lungs and using only a small percentage of their five-quart capacity. This poor breathing habit developed from several causes. First, many of us learned in childhood that good posture meant tucking in our stomachs and pushing out our chests. (Try that and see how it constricts the muscles that allow you to breathe.) A second cause for our shallow breathing is the mostly sedentary lives many of us lead. And third, accumulated tensions and worries, from which we all suffer to some extent, can cause the abdomen to be tight, which prevents us from inhaling deeply.

The result of our shallow, superficial breathing is that our bodies are deprived of both oxygen and prana (which is mainly supplied through the vehicle of oxygen) and we are prone to premature aging and the gradual deterioration of health.

## Self-Discovery Experience 7

### Are you really breathing?

After you've read this paragraph, close your eyes and observe your breathing. (It is not necessary to change it, just observe.) Is it shallow or deep? Slow or fast? Regular or irregular? How are you sitting? How does that affect your breathing? How do you feel right now? Sleepy and lazy? Alert and vigorous? Is the air around you warm or cool? Fresh or stuffy? Dry or moist? Sit still for a moment and get clear answers to these questions before reading on.

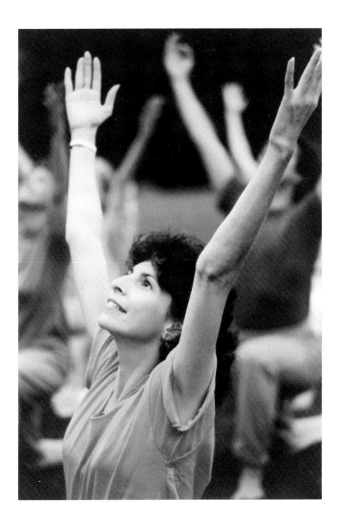

## Pranayama — the Science of Breath

Pranayama is the yogic science of gaining mastery over prana through special breathing techniques and through making breathing a more conscious process. Since all the functions of the body, voluntary and involuntary, are governed by prana, control of prana means improved functioning of all our organs and systems: respiratory, circulatory, digestive, glandular, and nervous. This results in greater resistance to disease, greater calmness, and more productivity.

Our mental processes, too, depend on the amount of prana we take in. The regular practice of pranayama dramatically increases mental clarity and concentration. Creative, intellectual, and intuitive capacities are greatly improved.

Pranayama also facilitates meditation because it establishes health and harmony of body and mind, allowing us to transcend both and enter into deeper states of consciousness. So pranayama is generally taught in yoga classes along with yoga postures.

Pranayama has a profound effect upon our emotions, as well as on our physical and mental states, because breathing corresponds closely to emotion. (Notice how you breathe when you are very angry or fearful, as compared to when you are relaxed and about to fall asleep.) Pranayama teaches us how to use breathing to transform negative or self-destructive emotions into positive growth.

Once we can maintain a relaxed breathing pattern when we are angry or tense, we are breaking a chain reaction. If our breathing pattern does not transmit a message of tension to our nervous system, the emotion will fail to leave its energy-draining stamp of stress on the body and mind. Usually, our emotions go unnoticed until they have become so overpowering that they are difficult to control.

Pranayama can also be extremely helpful in reducing smoking. People who smoke often report feeling tense and restless. Tension begins with the pattern of shallow breathing. So the need to smoke comes, in part, from the need to take in fuller, deeper breaths to relieve tension.

The act of smoking, however, does not fulfill the need for deeper breathing. Instead, it increases the negative cycle of shallow breathing, which creates more tension followed by more need to smoke.

With overeating, pranayama helps in much the same way. Overeating is a need of the mind and emotions, not of the stomach. Overeating temporarily relieves tension and unpleasant feelings such as loneliness, inadequacy, and insecurity. Yogic breathing helps to reduce the need to overeat by balancing the metabolism and calming the mind.

The regular practice of pranayama will lead to a state of relaxation and vigorous, holistic health by helping to balance and harmonize body, mind, and emotions. In this way, you are gaining the keys to life itself.

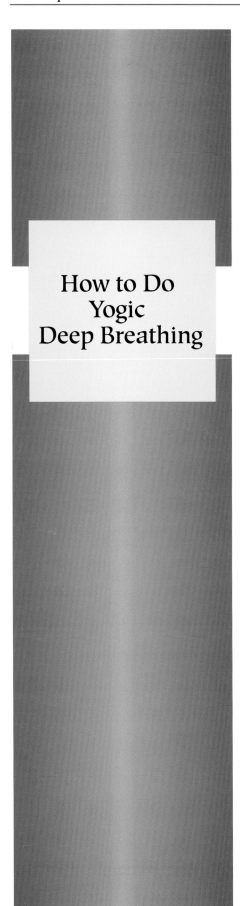

# How to Do Yogic Deep Breathing

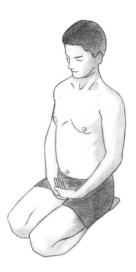

## Step 1. Abdominal Breathing

Stand, sit, or preferably lie in a very relaxed position. Breathe in slowly through your nose as you expand your abdomen. Imagine that you have a balloon inside that you are slowly inflating with each inhalation, and that causes the abdominal area to swell. Feel your diaphragm relaxing and being pushed down by the incoming air.

Breathe out slowly through your nose as you pull your abdominal muscles in, without straining, so that you press all of the air out of your lungs. Continue watching the abdomen rise as you breathe in and fall as you breathe out, until you establish a natural rhythm.

**HINT**: Place your hands on your abdomen just above the navel, with fingertips pointing toward each other and just touching. If you are breathing correctly, your hands will rise with your abdomen as you inhale and your fingertips will separate. As you exhale, they will touch again.

## Step 2. The "Sounding" Breath

After you are comfortable with abdominal breathing, you are ready to add the next step. In the back of the throat (where there is a small flap of flesh at the back of the soft palate) is the muscle that you use to gargle or snore. Imitate gargling and find the point where the sound originates.

Use that gargling muscle to draw the air into your lungs as you inhale and to control its outward flow as you exhale. Continue abdominal breathing through your nose. (Never breathe through the mouth.) You will hear the air being drawn through the throat much like the sound you hear when you press a large seashell to your ear.

That sound is not made by the voice, but by contraction of the throat. It is the sound you make through the mouth when you are fogging a mirror. You can learn to make this same sound while breathing in and out through the nose. Abdominal breathing is much easier when you inhale and exhale in this manner because you can control and extend the air flow.

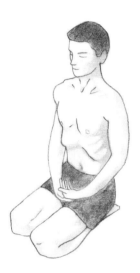

## Step 3. Full Yogic Breathing

When you are comfortable doing the abdominal breathing with the sound, you are ready to add the last step: Full Yogic Breathing. Follow the same steps listed for abdominal breathing. However, now imagine that your lungs are divided into two parts: the upper half (upper chest) and the lower half (the part you are already using in abdominal breathing).

As you inhale, fill the bottom half of the lungs (abdominal breathing) first and then continue to inhale, filling the top half. As you exhale, empty the top half of the lungs first and then empty the bottom half.

Imagine yourself filling a hot water bottle with water. The water enters and fills the bottom first and finally reaches the top. As you empty it, the water flows out first from the top and gradually down to the last drops remaining in the bottom, and the sides of the bottle contract together.

Posture is an important part of correct breathing. For your lungs to be free from compression and able to fill fully, your back should be straight but relaxed with shoulders down, back, and loose; your chin should be parallel to the ground and slightly tucked. Make sure your knees are unlocked and relaxed.

**BENEFITS:** Practice this Full Yogic Breathing as often as you can. It will provide more oxygenation of the blood, resulting in greater relaxation, better emotional balance and control, greater mental clarity and acuity, and greatly improved general health. Your lung capacity will gradually increase, so that you will be less easily winded by exertion. Even chronic lung and bronchial problems will be aided.

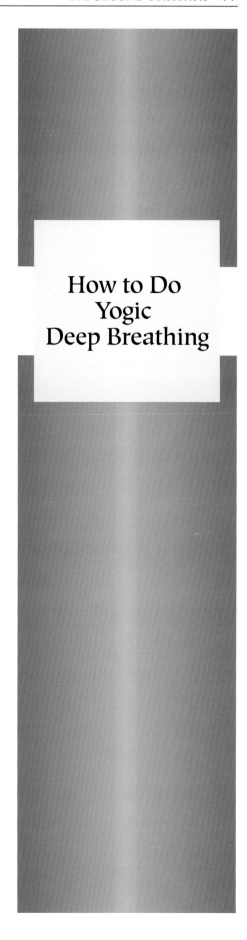

# How to Do Yogic Deep Breathing

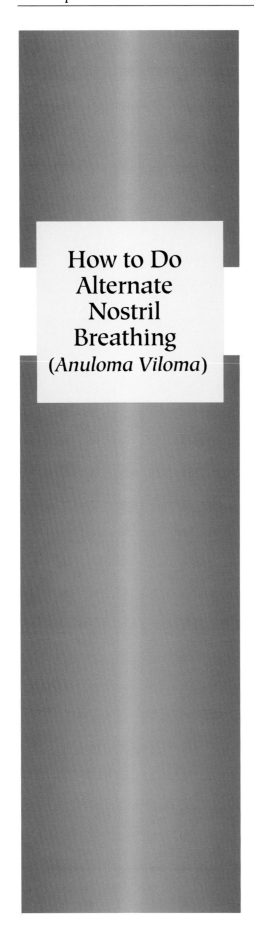

# How to Do Alternate Nostril Breathing (*Anuloma Viloma*)

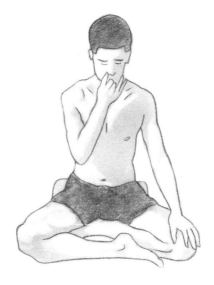

Alternate Nostril Breathing is the most powerful and beneficial of the various pranayamas (yogic breathing techniques). Its primary purpose is to soothe, purify, and strengthen the nervous system. Other benefits include developing control of the mind and emotions, increasing mental alertness, cleansing and opening the nasal passages, normalizing the metabolic processes, and helping to combat the overall detrimental effects of daily stress. Alternate Nostril Breathing also helps to establish a balanced breath pattern, believed by the ancient yogis to be important in maintaining overall health.

To do Alternate Nostril Breathing, you should be fairly comfortable with Yogic Deep Breathing (described above).

1. Assume a comfortable sitting position (in a chair or cross-legged on the floor) with your back straight. Sitting on a firm pillow or cushion may help you hold the position comfortably.

2. Using the right hand, press the index and middle fingers against the palm of the hand, holding out the thumb and last two fingers. The thumb will be used to close the right nostril and the last two fingers to close the left nostril. With practice this hand position will become quite comfortable.

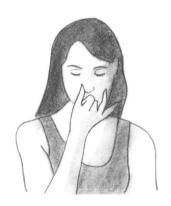 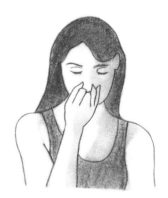 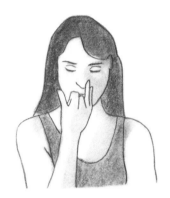

3. Using regular, slow Yogic Deep Breathing, close the right nostril and inhale through the left until the lungs are comfortably full. Then close off both nostrils and hold your breath. When you need to exhale, open the right nostril and exhale through that side alone. As soon as the lungs are completely empty, inhale again through the right, hold, then exhale again through the left. This comprises one round of Alternate Nostril Breathing (in left, out right, in right, out left). Practice it until you become accustomed to the pattern.

4. When you are comfortable with the pattern of Alternate Nostril Breathing, begin to count mentally, to time each inhalation, hold, and exhalation. At first, attempt to get them even and rhythmic by making each the same count: if you inhale to a count of four, then hold for four counts and exhale for four. As you improve, make the hold and exhalation longer and slower until the ratio is 1:4:2 (inhale for one count: hold four: exhale two). That is, if you inhale to a count of four, then hold for sixteen counts, and exhale for eight.

5. Begin by practicing for about five minutes at a time. Gradually increase your practice time until you are able to do Alternate Nostril Breathing for twenty minutes or more without rest. If you find yourself running out of breath, you need to exhale more completely each time. Soon you will be able to maintain the proper breathing ratio without counting.

# THE DIVINE DANCE OF KRIPALU YOGA
## by Yogi Amrit Desai

The word *yoga* means "unity." The great yogis devised many different techniques and branches of yoga and every one of those disciplines has only one purpose: to create internal harmony, peace, and unity. Any discipline of yoga that you practice must fulfill that purpose.

The real meaning of yoga is already known to you; it lies hidden within you as a potential. So the practice of yoga is only uncovering what is already there. Yogis believe that you are born divine, with a spiritual potential already present.

All you need to do is remove any physical, mental, or emotional blocks that are present, so that the radiant light of the soul may shine through and you can express its harmonious music. When the music of the soul begins to emanate, it is experienced as ecstasy and bliss. And with that comes true inner peace.

Sometimes you can practice the external form of yoga, and yet miss the spirit of yoga. For example, if you are practicing hatha yoga postures and your mind is creating internal doubts about the correctness of your postures, or you are experiencing indecision or questioning your flexibility or ability to practice yoga, then you are creating internal conflict while you are practicing the external form of yoga.

Most people are not conscious of this subtle part of the practice of yoga. Often the emphasis is so much on perfecting the external form that the spirit is lost. But the practice of yoga is not limited to its externally adopted form. The forms can be many; the purpose is always one. Yoga is not just a philosophy or theory. It is a practice that becomes a way of life. It encompasses everything we do, every moment of life. Only regular practice can reveal the true meaning of yoga. In the practice of Kripalu Yoga, body, mind, and prana work together to establish a deep inner sense of peace and harmony and gradually awaken higher consciousness.

In the first two stages of Kripalu Yoga practice, you learn how to perform yoga postures correctly, to control the breath, and to coordinate movement with breathing as you develop sensitivity and attunement to your body's sensations. While doing the postures, your mind is trained to focus on the subtle sensations of each bend, stretch, and twist.

As you breathe and enjoy the movement, you gradually become conscious of the parts of the body most actively engaged in the posture. And you focus on relaxing the areas that are not engaged, so that only the parts of the body that are needed are actually working.

By giving attention to these details, you may find that you are holding your breath, contracting un-

involved parts of the body, or struggling to achieve a certain position. All of those responses create unnecessary tension in the body. When you become aware of the tensions and how you create them, they begin to fall away without great effort.

Relaxed attention is the key to effective practice of Kripalu Yoga. The energy of the mind becomes focused naturally and effortlessly in the enjoyable sensations of movement and breath. This focusing of attention brings together your physical, emotional, and mental energies and establishes the groundwork of concentration skills necessary for the later stages of practice.

In the third stage of practicing Kripalu Yoga, your mind becomes sharp and focused. By performing yoga postures with extremely slow, meditative movements, you slow down the mind and induce the outgoing attention to be drawn inward. The mind becomes absorbed in the slow, flowing movements and gradually becomes a witness to the body's joyous and relaxing experience. The energy that is usually scattered and dissipated, as the mind attends to the ever-changing stimuli of the senses, is now totally focused inward. The focused mind serves as a bridge between the internal world and the external world, between spirit and matter.

In the fourth stage, you achieve intense concentration through the processes of visualization (mental images) and affirmation (positive mental suggestions). Using visualization and affirmation while performing yoga postures helps the body release unconscious patterns of tension and contraction. In some postures and movements, holding tension may have become so habitual and mechanical that you are constantly creating undesirable muscular contractions in the body.

The powerful tools of visualization and affirmation can alter long-established patterns in the brain that may have greatly limited your patterns of movement and altered your structural alignment. Energy is naturally drawn to the part of the body where the attention is focused. This energy, working in harmony with the mind, frees the body for its most effective, efficient, and graceful expression.

For example, the spinal twist posture (*Matsyendrasana*) tones and strengthens the spinal muscles and nerves. It is an excellent posture to help correct curvature of the spine (scoliosis), which is often created by an imbalance in the major back muscles that support correct posture. In this posture, the back is extended and lengthened while twisting.

To increase the extension, you can visualize prana as a rope of light running from the base of the spine to an imaginary pulley just above the crown of the head. You can see the cord of light effortlessly pulling the body into a straighter position. The body will automatically begin to straighten in response to that mental image. If you add the simple affirmation "My back muscles are relaxing and lengthening," the body receives an even stronger message to release its habitual muscular tensions.

In the fifth stage of Kripalu yoga practice, postures, breathing, and other tension-releasing *kriyas* (involuntary cleansing and cathartic activities) are performed spontaneously and effortlessly. In this final stage, body movements are prompted by prana. Yoga postures occur spontaneously as the innate wisdom of prana moves the body. The mind remains in an objective witness state, observing the movement rather than directing it. Everything that has been learned from books, traditions, and authorities about formal yoga postures and breathing exercises drops away.

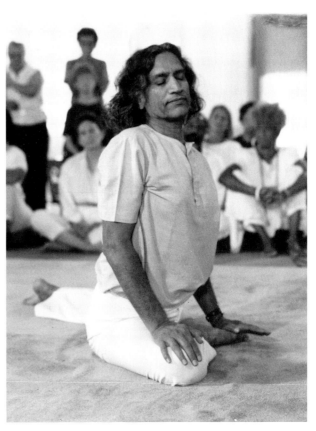

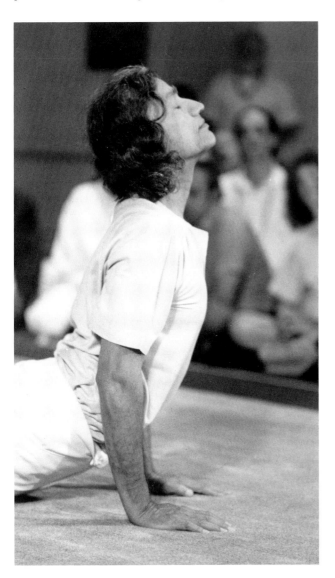

Ultimately there is only one book to read for the practice of yoga: the book of your body, and only one authority: your inner guidance. You'll find your body creating new postures and new sequences each day, as you feel the intense signals of prana urging you into intuitive movement. The body begins to move, turn, and twist automatically, directed by its own inner wisdom, while the mind watches as a relaxed spectator. Because the inner energy orchestrates and choreographs these movements, they are precisely and finely tuned to your needs. Your attention is automatically drawn inward, and concentration and meditation emerge naturally. Kripalu Yoga then becomes an effortless, rhythmic, and balanced flow of postures and breath that produces inner stillness. The flow is guided from within in a meditative way that gives a timeless quality to the movement. As you flow smoothly from one posture to another, the inner stillness progressively grows until you become completely absorbed in the inner music of movements created by the harmony of mind, body, and prana. Experienced in this way, yoga postures have a totally new dimension. They become a meditation in motion, a prayer without words.

# The Five Stages of Kripalu Yoga

Yogi Amrit Desai has systematized Kripalu Yoga into five stages, each of which highlights a particular aspect of the practice. Together they correspond to the eight stages of the complete practice of Hatha and Raja Yogas delineated by Patanjali in his *Yoga Sutras*.

In classical yoga the eight stages are practiced sequentially; in Kripalu yoga they are experienced simultaneously. Although each stage focuses on one aspect of the discipline and may be considered a prerequisite to the stage that follows, the unique quality of Kripalu Yoga is that the experience of the Stage Five spontaneous posture flow or Meditation in Motion is available from the very beginning, which makes the practice of the early stages very rich and compelling.

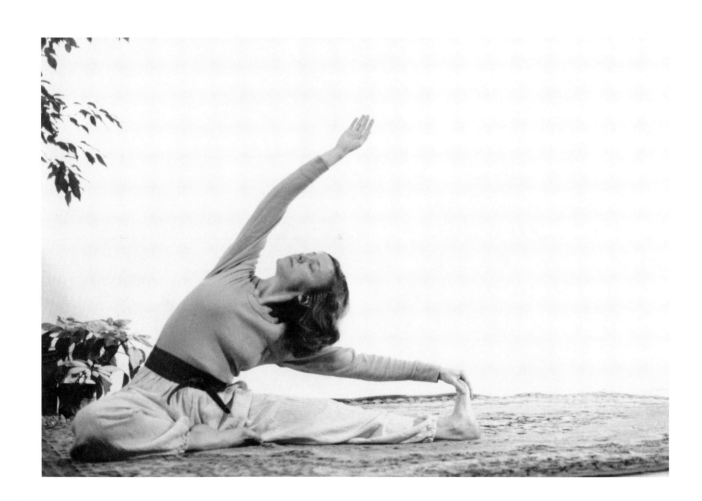

### Stage One —
### Mastering the Posture

At this level, you learn to perform the postures, doing them at your own comfort level. When you have learned how to enter, hold, and release the postures, you move on to the other stages, but, in reality, perfecting the postures continues over many years as the body becomes more flexible.

### Stage Two —
### Coordinating the Breathing
### with the Posture

Here the focus is on synchronizing deep yogic breathing with every movement: inhaling as you unfold and stretch, exhaling as you bend over or curl up.

### Stage Three —
### Holding and Concentrating

In this stage, you practice moving even more slowly and remaining in the posture for a longer period of time, while concentrating the energy of your attention on the parts of the body that are particularly being affected.

### Stage Four —
### Creative Visualization and Affirmation

Now as you direct your inner energy (prana) consciously to the parts of the body being benefited by the posture, you deliberately and willfully increase those benefits by visualizing relaxation and healing energy in the form of light and heat flowing to that area.

### Stage Five —
### Spontaneous Posture Flow

The purpose of the first four stages of physical and mental discipline is to help you get more in touch with your prana and to facilitate its free flow throughout your body. Now, you cease to direct your movements with your mind and allow them to become spontaneous and unchoreographed.

As prana is allowed to take over, the mind relaxes into simply witnessing what becomes a meditation in motion. First the mind learned to become an agent of prana, rather than of the individualized ego. Now the mind is gently set aside as the inner wisdom of the universal life force orchestrates the movements of your body directly, just as it does those of a newborn baby or a cat stretching after sleep.

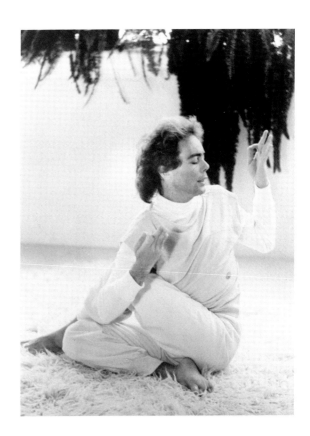

## STOP!

How aware are you of your body messages right now? How are you feeling? Is there tension, stiffness, or tiredness in any part of your body? Do you need to get up and stretch? Take some deep breaths? Relax your shoulders? Rest your eyes? Rest your mind? Close your eyes for a minute and take some long, slow, deep breaths to enable you to get in touch with your experience. Then respond to what your body is asking you to do.

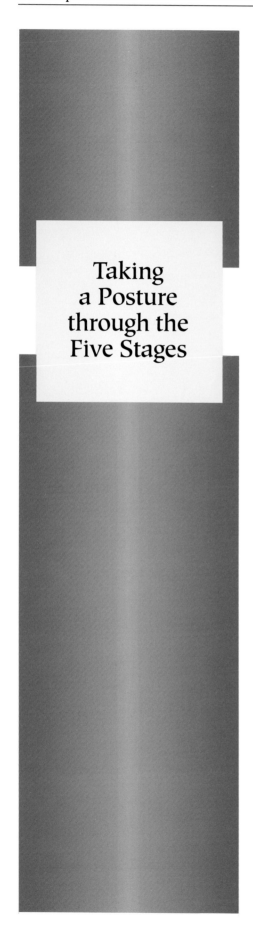

## Taking a Posture through the Five Stages

### STAGE 1:
### Mastering the Posture

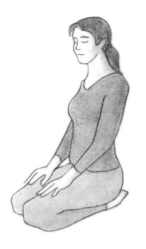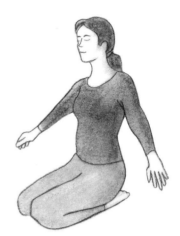

### STAGE 2:
### Coordinating Breathing and Movement

**NOTE:** We've combined Stages 1 and 2 of Kripalu Yoga in these directions for easy following.

1. To begin, kneel with hands on your thighs, palms down. Sit straight, but relaxed. Close your eyes. Take slow, deep breaths through the nose, breathing into the abdomen fully. Take a moment to relax. Concentrate your attention and energy on your body.

2. Inhaling slowly, raise your hands up from the thighs, and let them float very slowly behind your hips. Imagine that the inhaled breath is moving them through space.

3. Holding the breath for a moment, interlock your fingers, pull the shoulder blades together, and drop the head slightly back.

4. Gently exhale, very slowly. While exhaling, begin to bend forward, raising your arms and interlocked hands over your head. Bend forward until your forehead or chin rests on the floor.

5. Breathe slowly and deeply using Yogic Deep Breathing while holding. Hold as is comfortable for you; in the beginning, it may be a very short time. Do not strain.

6. As you gently inhale, rise slowly up again, leading with your arms. Rise until your head is erect and your hands are behind your hips. Keep your shoulders relaxed and down.

7. Exhaling fully, lightly release the fingers and let the arms float on the exhaling breath back to your thighs. Rest for a moment, still taking slow, yogic breaths, and feel the effects of the Yoga Mudra in your body and state of mind.

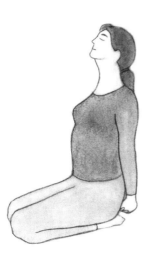

## STAGE 4:
## Creative Affirmation and Visualization

Still coordinating breath with movement, activate the life energy or prana within yourself through this stage of creative visualization. Read the following visualization to yourself several times. Then practice the Yoga Mudra, carrying the visualization into your experience.

Gently and slowly begin to move through the Yoga Mudra. As your arms and body move, feel that they are moving not through your conscious will, but through the rhythm and power of your breath. Imagine that you are moving under water: slowly, gracefully, and silently. While you hold the posture, feel a deep peace descend over your mind and body. Watch the overstimulated, misused nerves and organs of your abdomen relax. Feel their gratitude for this welcome release from tension. Complete the posture with calm resolve to carry this physical and mental tranquility through your day's activities.

## STAGE 3:
## Holding and Concentrating

Close your eyes; become still and calm. Visualize yourself from this place of stillness moving effortlessly through the posture. Then repeat the Yoga Mudra as guided in Stages 1 and 2. Keep your mind focused, absorbed in the body's movement. Try to increase your holding time in the bending forward position. Guideline: five to ten seconds in the beginning, gradually increasing to three minutes duration. As you hold the position, continue with slow, deep yogic breaths. Let yourself be absorbed in the holding and allow the posture to happen; do not strain or force.

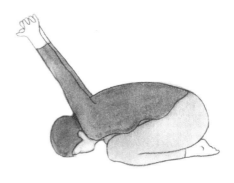

## STAGE 5:
## Incorporating the Posture into a Spontaneous Flow

To get the feel of a posture flow, sit quietly for a moment in the completed Yoga Mudra, then, following the prompting of your body, move into another, perhaps complementary, posture and take it through the five stages.

Don't be concerned if at first the messages regarding the next posture in a flow seem to come from your mind: prana is simply using the vehicle of communication that is available. As you are able to relax the mind and trust that the body will flow from posture to posture with perfect wisdom, prana will begin to move you without the mind having to play its role of intermediary.

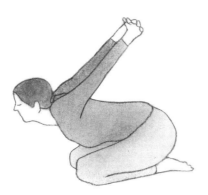

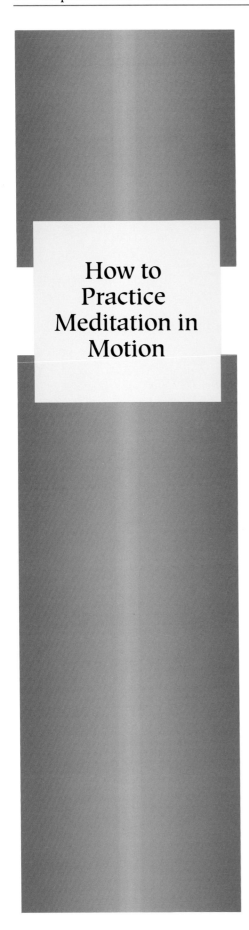

## How to Practice Meditation in Motion

### A Beginning Exercise

Before you begin to do a Kripalu Yoga posture flow, try this very simple exercise. It is so easy that anyone of any age or physical condition can do it, yet it gives a deep and real experience of the flow of Kripalu Yoga. It should take about ten minutes:

1. Choose a quiet, secluded place and dim the lights. Begin by sitting in a cross-legged position on the floor (or if that is really uncomfortable, sit in a straight-backed chair with your feet on the floor in front of you). Keep your spine straight and hold your neck and back in alignment, with chin parallel to the floor and tucked in slightly. Close your eyes and relax your body.

2. Slowly rotate your head in both directions to release any neck tension. Shrug your shoulders a few times and rotate them up and back. To release any tension in your hands and arms, make fists with both hands and squeeze as hard as you can. Hold for a moment, then relax your hands. Shake your hands and fingers as if something was stuck on the ends of the fingers and you wanted to shake it off. Then allow your hands to relax completely as you place them on your knees, palms facing upward.

3. Begin to take long, slow, deep, and uniform yogic breaths. Allow the deep breaths to relax your body and calm your mind even more.

4. After several minutes of breathing, focus your attention on your solar plexus. Visualize pranic energy as a warm, luminous, liquid light glowing in the solar plexus. See or feel it clearly.

5. Begin to picture that energy flowing up through your chest, down your arms, and into your hands. Concentrate on directing all the energy into the hands. Actually visualize your hands and fingers filling with light.

6. Continue to concentrate on the energy flowing into your hands until you feel them wanting to rise up from your knees. Allow that to happen. If your hands remain on your lap, you can consciously lift them gently off your knees and then allow the movement to continue on its own. Do not expect anything specific to happen. The key to this exercise is to concentrate on your prana and observe its workings.

   Let your hands continue to float upward, as you keep your elbows at your sides, and let them move toward your face in an extremely slow, almost invisible, movement. You may feel that your hands are being moved without your conscious will; that is an experience of prana.

   As your hands reach your face, allow your fingers to move gently across it according to patterns that arise spontaneously from within. Feel that as your fingertips move across your face they are discharging prana, which deeply relaxes the muscles and erases lines.

7. Now allow your hands to drift back down to their original position, letting the movement be extremely slow, almost invisible. When your hands have come to rest on your knees, remain in a sitting position with your eyes closed for as long as you wish. When you are ready, gently open your eyes and allow the muscles of the body to stretch. Experience the rejuvenation, the healing, that has happened within you.

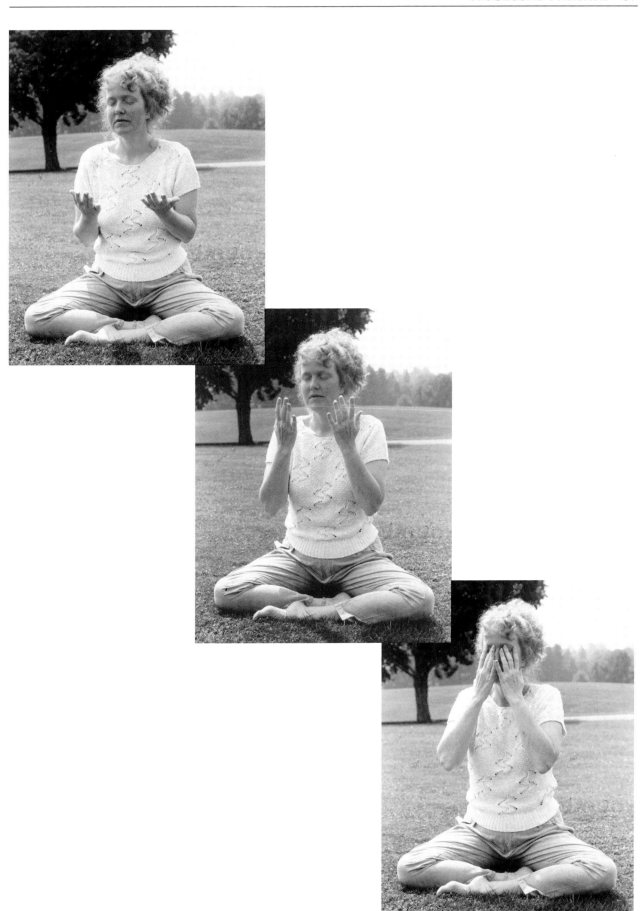

## Self-Discovery Experience 8

**Rediscovering the past through your body**

### Awareness

After reading these instructions, close your eyes and relax, allowing the answers to come to you spontaneously from the feelings in your body rather than from the thoughts in your mind. Let this be an experiential trip into the past for you.

1. Going over your whole body, part by part, try to get in touch with its personal history. Recall incidents in the past that particularly involved that part of your body. It might be a time when you were injured, or when you became especially conscious of how much you depended on it.

   For example, you might get in touch with the time or times that you fell off your bike as a child and grazed your knee. Or the time you broke your wrist, had your arm in a cast, and couldn't do the things you wanted to do. Really get in touch with how you felt at that time.

2. Also remember the times when a particular part of your body pleased you or surprised you. For instance, recall how good you felt about your legs one day when you ran a race faster than ever before, or when someone complimented you on your healthy feet or good posture.

3. Jot down for yourself, as you go, the words and images that come to you, or make drawings if that feels more appropriate.

### Acceptance

4. What have you learned about your body that you didn't know before? Write down all the thoughts, feelings, and emotions that came to you as you did this exercise.

### Adjustment

5. Write down some specific things that you see you might do to benefit from what you have just become aware of and what you have learned from that awareness. For example, you might realize that you need to work at making your arms and shoulders more flexible, after remembering a time when you learned to hold them rigidly as a result of an experience that had a profound impact on you.

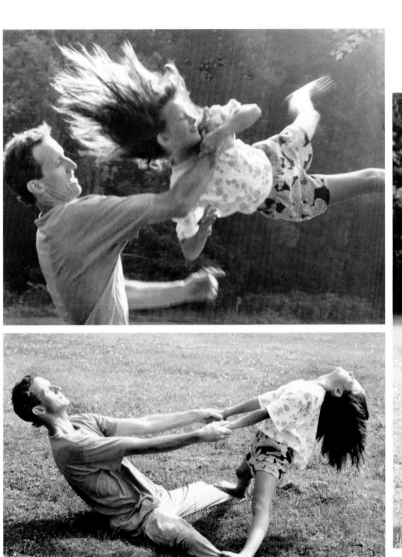

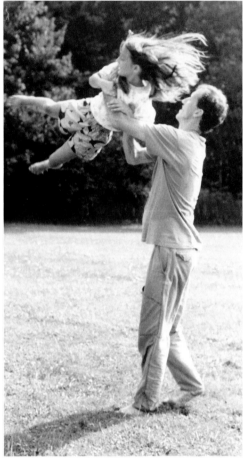

# Running

## Why Run?

Modern medicine has compiled an impressive list of physical benefits that come from daily exercise, especially from swimming, cycling, and running. Of these three, running is by far the most frequently and most conveniently practiced, and its benefits are dramatic on mental and emotional levels as well as the physical.

The physical benefits of running are many. Your body soon begins to lose excess weight. Your muscles become compact and toned all over your body. Your skin tightens and takes on a rosy glow of health. Your capacity for work of all kinds is increased. Your movements become quicker, more energetic, and fluid.

By stabilizing and physically purifying the body through running, your emotions also become more stable and less subject to reaction and irritation. Through focusing on the physical realities of running, your mind becomes more steady and less restless. Running (especially longer distance running) is a wonderful means to forget the everyday cares of the world as you become absorbed in the body, the fresh air, and the beautiful scenery.

## Who Should — and Shouldn't — Run?

Running is not a difficult sport, but there are a few beginning awarenesses that may save you physical discomfort and discouragement as you begin your running program.

If you are out of condition, over thirty-five years of age, or have a specific physical problem that may be affected by running, a medical checkup would be your first step. If possible, select a doctor who is also a runner, or at least is somewhat sympathetic to its benefits. Some conditions that may warrant special medical guidance in running are advanced arthritis, heart disease and hypertension, some orthopedic problems, and diabetes.

Men over thirty-five should have checkups even if they feel they are in good health and physical condition. A stress electrocardiogram (measuring the heart's reaction to physical effort) is recommended by many running experts and doctors.

Some physical conditions, such as those involving the heart, may be improved through a sensible program of running, but such a program should never be attempted without a doctor's supervision.

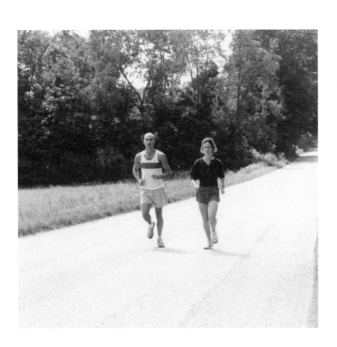

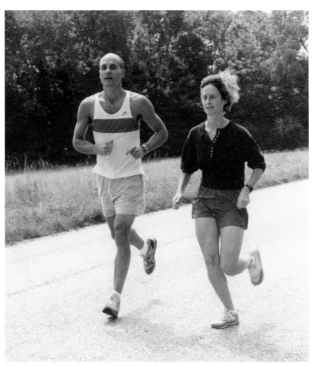

## How Do I Start?

If you are out of condition, begin gradually and gently. Remember how long it took for you to get out of condition and accept the fact that you cannot change it overnight. Begin by practicing some stretching exercises each day (perhaps using the yoga postures described in this book), followed by a brisk walk.

When you find you can walk for fifteen to twenty minutes without tiring, add intervals of slow running to your walk. Run slowly and gently until you feel yourself begin to tire or strain, then walk until you are ready to run again. Repeat these intervals of running and walking as often as you can with comfort. Gradually your intervals of jogging will increase and, in time, the need to walk should disappear.

Do not worry about the distance you cover, especially if you are a beginner. If you need a challenge, set a length of time, rather than a distance, to remain out (twenty to thirty minutes is a good beginning) and gradually increase it as you feel able. However, do not push yourself too far, too fast; it should be enjoyable. To see whether or not you are pushing, check if you can hold a conversation as you run. If you get out of breath, you need to slow down!

## The Microcosm of Running — A Personal Experience

*Easily moving through the space of a gentle countryside, I feel revitalizing cool air pouring in and out: I'm running with me. Like many runners, I have always experienced a peaceful and deep sense of myself during a run. But my experience with yoga has brought new benefits.*

*When I run now, I gain deeper knowledge and insight into my inner world. I see only too clearly my overall attitudes mirrored in reactions to hills, barking dogs, rainstorms, and sunrises. Everything becomes symbolic.*

*When my mind hits a snag while running, I immediately recognize the tension I'm feeling because it makes my breath labored and my movement less free. When I'm four or five miles from home, I have no choice but to deal with whatever is inside of me and drop it by the wayside. So I've realized more and more that what I see as problems must really be very insignificant if I can drop them so easily!*

*There's no overlooking the numerous physical benefits of running. But more important, I've come to see that by coming in touch with true joy at least once a day, my whole life has just naturally changed for the better.*

*Joy creates a thirst for more, which has made me aware of my diet and use of energy. I can feel the benefits of proper eating so clearly each morning as I head off over the hills.*

*Lastly, I've seen that the happier my body is, the happier my mind is, and the happier my spirit is — an amazing cycle that wonderfully feeds and perpetuates itself.*

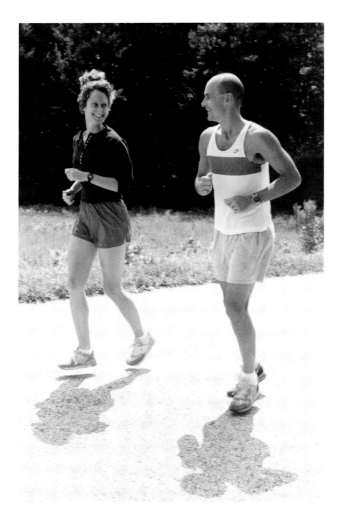

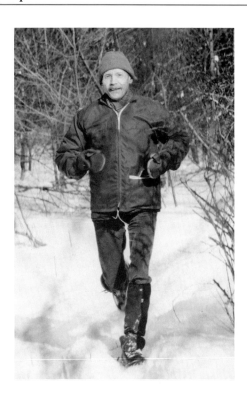

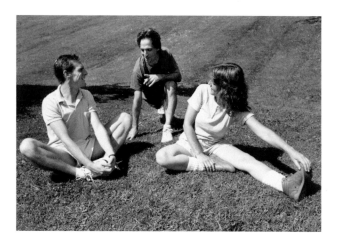

## Some Kripalu Hints on Running

Two things that the Kripalu Approach emphasizes when you run are being gentle with yourself — never straining or forcing — and making it an internal experience of yourself and your body, rather than a competition or test of endurance.

Always give your body time to warm up at the beginning of a run by starting slowly. That allows the blood vessels to expand, the blood to circulate more freely, and enough oxygen to be carried to the muscles for aerobic combustion (burning blood sugar for fuel in the presence of oxygen). Starting too fast causes anaerobic (without oxygen) combustion, which builds up toxic wastes in the muscles, such as ptomaine and lactic acid, and results in pain and strain.

Some anaerobic or resistance running is beneficial for accelerated burning of fat and strengthening of muscles but it should be done only after the body is thoroughly warmed up. Anaerobic running means running without burning oxygen in the cells, and is thus more demanding on the body.

Concentrate on your breathing, making it deep and regular; it will carry you along.

Focus your attention on your body awareness and inner experience, rather than on how far or how fast you can run.

Do it regularly: with regular practice the body will get slimmer, firmer, and more able to handle stress on all levels.

Do wind-down stretching exercises at the end of your run for at least five minutes.

## What Equipment Do I Need?

**SHOES:**
Shoes are the only major purchase you will need to make to begin running — and the most important. Proper shoes will save you needless discomfort and even injury, so take time to select them well.

Much has been written on the subject of choosing running shoes. A little research will yield a flood of valuable information. Then let your experience complete the process by visiting a number of stores and trying on a variety of brands and types. Be sure to wear the socks you plan to run in. Take your time.

Check each pair for fit, comfort, light weight, and flexibility. Are the soles durable, yet cushioned to absorb shock? Is there enough room for the toes and support for the heels?

**CLOTHING:**
Expensive running outfits may be enjoyable, if you can afford them, but they are not a necessity. Simple items of clothing that you may already own or that can be purchased inexpensively will suffice. What is important is comfort and suitability to the weather.

In hot weather, clothing should be minimal. Nylon and lycra are very popular for their light weight. Light colors or white will reflect heat and a light cap will keep the sun from your head.

In cold weather do not dress too warmly. Allow for the body heat you will be generating. Layers of clothing will help to keep you warm, as the body heat warms the air between the layers. Also, you may want to remove a few layers as you get too hot (but be sure to put them back on as soon as you stop, or you will get chilled).

A windbreaker (usually nylon is preferred) is very useful because it is lightweight but keeps in the body heat. A warm cap is also advisable, since eighty percent of the body's heat escapes through the head.

# Walking

## The Gentle Alternative

For some ages and body types, walking may be a more appropriate form of aerobic exercise than running. Like running, walking can be done almost anytime, anywhere and offers the same physical benefits as running, while having the advantage of being easier on some parts of the body, such as the knees and lower back. And you get a better view of the scenery! By aerobic walking we don't, of course, mean strolling, as pleasant and healthy as that activity is. Walking done for aerobic exercise is only slightly slower than jogging.

## Kripalu Hints on the Aerobic Walk

Do some stretching exercises before setting out, then begin with a slow walking pace. Walk with your head erect, your shoulders relaxed, and your pelvis tucked under your torso. Gradually build up speed, maintaining a heel-to-toe movement in each step.

Bring your arms into the exercise, bending them at the elbows and swinging them in rhythm with your step. You'll find that you can develop a flowing, complementary motion between your arms and legs.

Walk at a pace that challenges your body without straining, slowing down and speeding up in response to its signals.

Be sure to stay within a range of pacing that enables you to breathe deeply and rhythmically without shortness of breath.

## Big Results for Not-So-Big Efforts

You'll be amazed at your progress. Within a few days, you will begin to experience the physical, mental, and emotional benefits that only aerobic exercise brings. And it's safe, painless, and fun!

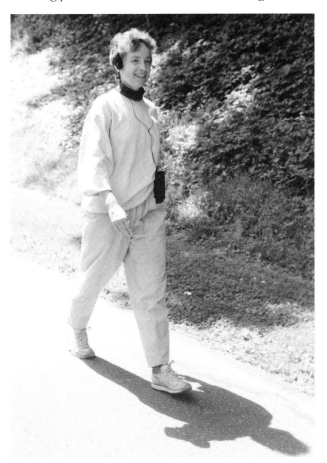

**STOP!**

How aware are you of your body messages right now? How are you feeling? Is there tension, stiffness, or tiredness in any part of your body? Do you need to get up and stretch? Take some deep breaths? Relax your shoulders? Rest your eyes? Rest your mind? Close your eyes for a minute and take some long, slow, deep breaths to enable you to get in touch with your experience. Then respond to what your body is asking you to do.

# Self-Discovery Experience 9

## Body mapping

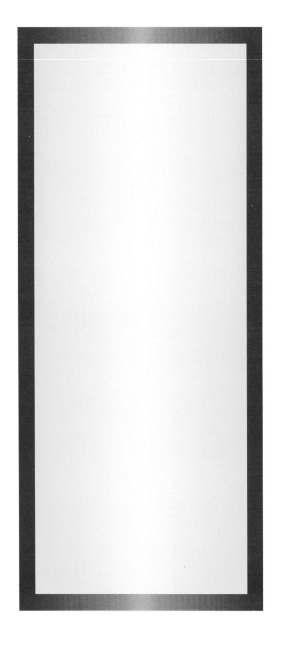

### Awareness

1. Sit quietly and get in touch with your body. Be aware of how it feels at this moment; experience each inner movement, every change in rhythm. Begin to see your body in vivid colors. Give a color and shape to each part and organ, even if you do not know technically what it is, where it is, or what it looks like. Use your creative imagination to visualize it.

2. Open your eyes, take some colored crayons and, without beginning to think too much about it, start to draw a map of your own body. Allow the map to illustrate your feelings about your body, as well as how you experience it in an objective way. For example, if you really like and feel good about one particular part of your body, try to draw/color in that feeling. If a part gives you trouble, see if you can depict that in some way.

### Acceptance

3. Take a long, hard look at your map. See what it tells you about yourself and your body image and perceptions. Look at it very objectively, as if it had been drawn by someone else. See what you can learn from your map about your unconscious feelings about your body, as opposed to the habitual ways you think about it.

### Adjustment

4. Now decide what all this means to you. Is there some adjustment you need to make in your image of yourself? Is there a disparity you'd like to remedy between what you consciously think of your body and your unconscious image of yourself? For example, do you see that you have drawn the top of your body out of proportion to the bottom? Does that mean that you need to pay more attention to what is going on in the lower part of your body?

5. Write some specific ways you can be aware of and experiment with what you have just learned about yourself that you didn't know before.

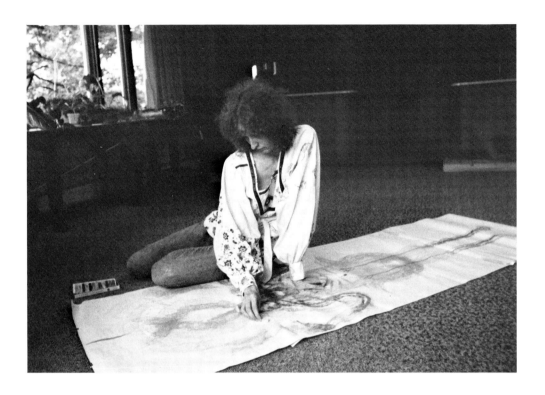

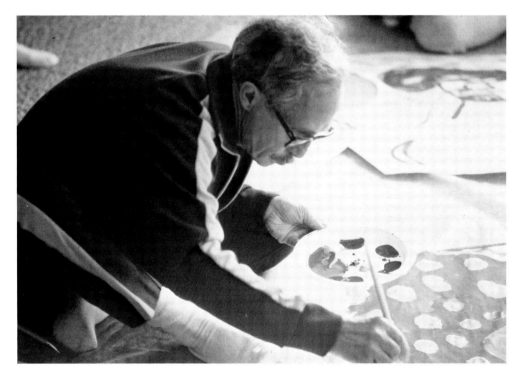

# Massage:
# A Helping Hand to Free Up Your Prana

Massage is a time-honored method of relieving muscular distress. It was used by the ancient Greeks and Romans, and the Egyptians before them, to relieve physical pain and injury and make the body supple. But it plays an even more fundamental role in holistic health.

The Kripalu Approach teaches that physical tension and stiffness do not just stem from physical activity or inactivity. The body is actually a mirror reflecting our mind and emotions, so that physical tension is a result of what we are experiencing mentally and emotionally.

Throughout our lives we are exposed to potentially tension-producing situations and this mental tension is expressed in our bodies. Because this is often unconscious, we do not take steps to dissipate the tension and it gradually builds up over the years.

Generally we experience tension in the same parts of our bodies habitually (neck and shoulders, forehead, lower back, abdomen), and over a period of time, without our realizing it, those patterns of tension become permanently lodged in our bodies as energy blocks.

Visualize the energy of water blocked by a twist in the garden hose. That kind of block affects our health, our posture, our minds, and emotions — our whole way of being in the world. Tension inhibits our ability to experience the full freedom of body and mind that is the essence of holistic health.

The cornerstone of the Kripalu Approach to holistic health is attuning ourselves to prana energy, and the relaxation of physical and mental tension is a prerequisite to that. Massage is a key way to get in touch with prana because it can dissipate tensions lodged in the muscles, not just in the preceding hours or days, but over a lifetime.

Often during a massage, recipients will reexperience a painful situation of many years before as they feel the physical release of tension during the massage of a particular part of the body. They report afterwards that they feel sure they have been released from the stored emotional trauma as well as the physiological one.

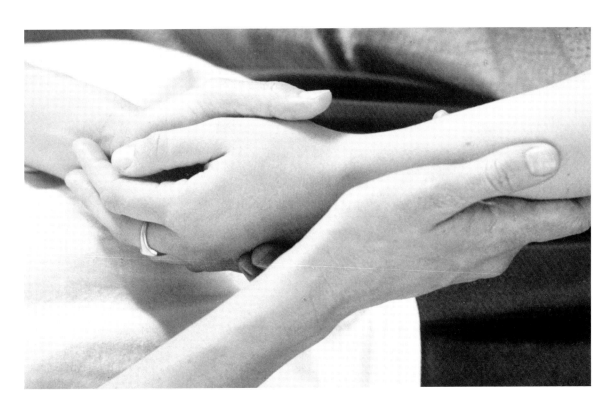

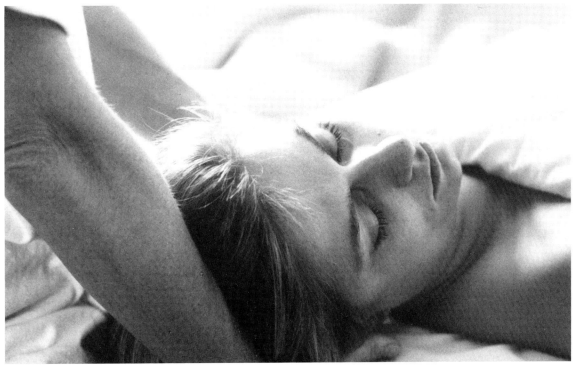

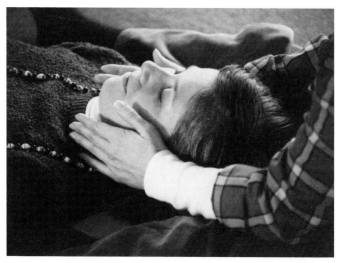

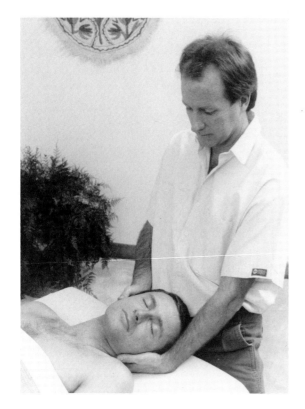

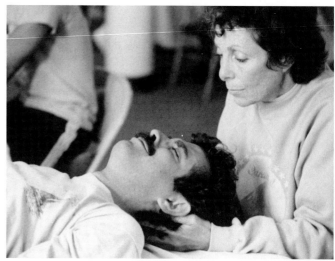

## Specific Therapeutic Benefits of Massage

In physiological terms, what happens in the course of a thorough, therapeutic, deep body massage is this:

The circulation improves as the blood vessels dilate from the warmth of friction.

Wastes and toxins are released and eliminated from tense muscles by the pressure.

Muscle tone is improved so the muscular system functions better.

An increased flow of nutrients to the muscles is facilitated by the improved circulation and relaxation of the muscle fibers.

Psychologically, people who receive a massage begin to enjoy their bodies more — to feel better about the body as it feels better to them — and this positive attitude in turn produces greater health and vitality.

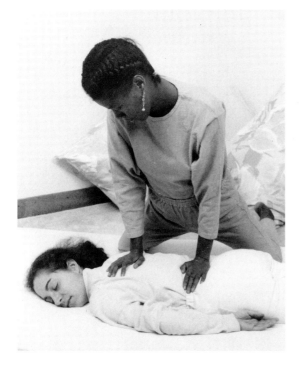

## Massage as Meditation — A Personal Experience

*My Kripalu massage was an experience of being totally one with what was happening, one with my prana. After a few initial shared words of explanation and trust, my eyes closed and I relaxed into just feeling.*

*It is so rare for most of us simply to feel our bodies for an extended period of time, without judging, thinking, or commenting. In this meditative massage, my mind was still active, but secondary, just a monotonous background voice that kept receding and fading.*

*Effortlessly, my consciousness followed the firm, yet gentle fingers, discovering my body with them. I had been fasting and taking enemas and had just had a sauna, so many of my customary pain and tension places (like neck and shoulders) were relatively loose and pain-free, to my surprise.*

*But I discovered others that amazed me. My legs, for example, felt fine until those probing fingers discovered the buried tensions and blocks in buttocks and thighs and calf muscles—and the soles of my feet. Those strange re-flex mirrors of the body felt like a burning iron was being run along them, yet it was only a thumb!*

*At those times, I breathed deeply and slowly into the pain, as I have learned to do, and was astonished to see how far I have come in dealing with pain in the past three years of Kripalu Yoga. I don't fear or fight it any more. I really know how to go with it, to ride its waves like a surfer, and to embrace it simply as a part of my experience. With my acceptance, pain has become transformed.*

*What I am calling pain in the massage is not, of course, like real pain from injury. The acute sensation for which I have no other word than pain is really an exquisite suffer-ing because I know it is releasing buried pains of tension and blockage.*

*The most amazing and beautiful thing in the massage was the pacing. The hands of the masseuse moved slowly and constantly across my muscles, always flowing at the same steady pace and pressure and always synchronized with an audible, deep breathing that in itself was deeply relaxing to hear, like the murmur of the tide on a distant seashore.*

*This massage was indeed Kripalu Yoga Meditation in Motion, just as much as a Hatha Yoga posture flow, and thus had the same effect of drawing me into deep, effort-less meditation. It was a unique and wonderful experience.*

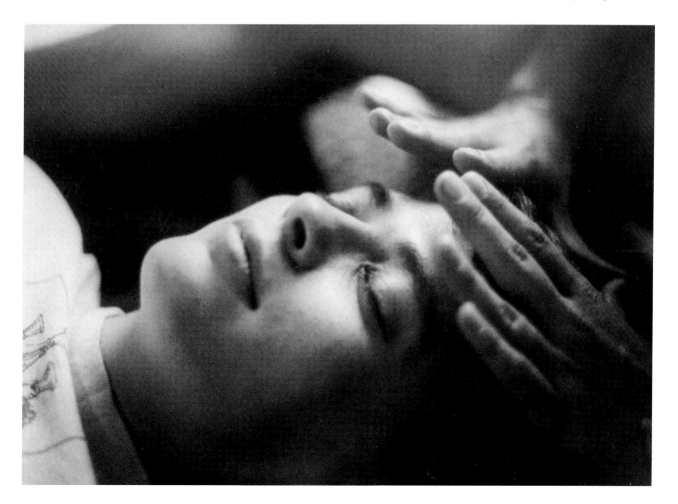

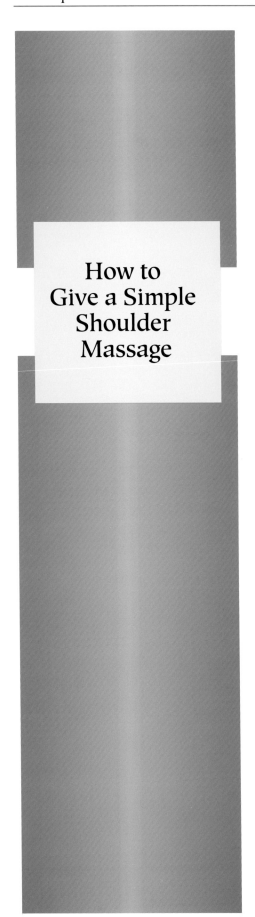

# How to Give a Simple Shoulder Massage

Attitude is the key to the Kripalu method of massage. Anyone can learn the mechanics and physical moves of massage, but a truly loving, giving, meditative approach makes all the difference between mere physical relief and the deep sense of peace and well-being afforded by a Kripalu massage. The key points are these:

Begin with a relaxed and loving attitude, secure in the knowledge that however little you may know intellectually about technique, your prana will flow from you to the recipient if you're relaxed and loving.

Know that giving truly is receiving. After you give your first massage, that will be your own experience. Because your prana flows more freely when you are deeply concentrated on giving another a massage and because of the satisfaction you will feel at giving them the gift of relaxation, you too will feel deeply relaxed and energized.

Really BE THERE for your friend. Your prana flows immediately to where your attention is, so if you concentrate fully on your hands, the healing force of prana will work through them. You will feel them become very warm and tingling with prana energy as you work.

Make the massage a meditative flow, a slow-motion dance. Breathe slowly and deeply, in harmony with your movements. As you become familiar with the movements, try working with your eyes closed.

Visualize the prana as warm, radiant liquid light flowing into the parts of the body you are massaging. Ask your friend to try to visualize it with you.

Use firm, strong pressure. That communicates confidence and also feels better to the recipient. Keep your hands constantly touching his/her body to keep the energy contact.

Feel as if the massage is happening to your own body, so that you know exactly where and how to touch.

## Step by Step Instructions

This simple neck and shoulder massage is most easily done with the recipient sitting on the floor, cross-legged or kneeling. Those with older or less flexible bodies may be more comfortable sitting on a chair with their feet flat on the floor.

The massage has infinite variations — let PRANA lead you! Draw on your own experience of what eases tension and be guided by your inner sense of where tension is accumulated.

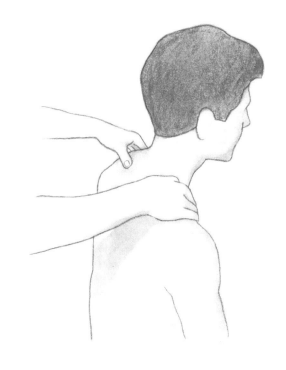

1.  Place your palms firmly on your friend's shoulders and make deep contact. Take a few deep breaths and ask him/her to do so as well.

2.  Smooth down the arms and the entire back with light, gentle strokes. Use your whole hand.

3.  Do a brisk circular rub with the heel of your hand down the whole of the back. (Divide the back mentally into vertical sections and do one at a time, top to bottom.) Then rub the arms.

4.  Shoulder Kneading: Keep your palm on the back of the shoulder as much as possible and knead the large muscle along the top of the shoulder by using your fingers (held together and hooked over in front of the shoulder, taking care not to press directly on the collar bone). Imagine you are kneading bread. Use the ball of your hand to push the muscle into the heel of your hand and your thumb. The emphasis is on creating a smooth wave-like motion.

    Let your thumbs reach down between the shoulder blades to work that area, keeping your fingers still over the shoulders. Also let your thumb follow the curve of the shoulder blade, outlining the top and side closest to the spine.

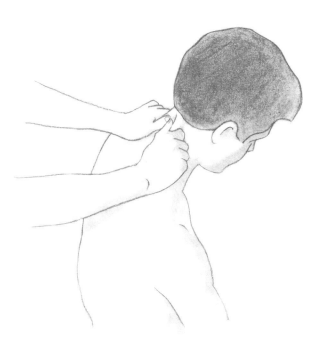

5.  Lift the large shoulder muscle between your thumb and fingers. Press in and hold it briefly at tense spots, asking your friend to take deep breaths while you hold.

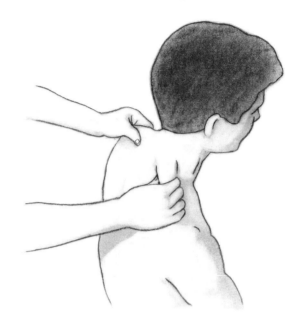

6. Use your thumbs to press directly down on the shoulder muscle in a line beginning at the "V" where the collar bone and shoulder blade meet at the outer edge of the shoulder and work in toward the spine. There are points in this area that are VERY effective tension releasers. They are also likely to be very tender, so be gentle until you determine how hard to press.

   Good firm pressure is most effective. Ask your friend to take deep breaths while you hold the points. You will get better pressure if you stand on your knees. Ask for feedback as to whether you've found the right spot.

7. Pinch the muscles that run up either side of the spine at the neck between your thumb and first two fingers, working up the neck with a circling motion. This is very relaxing!

8. Do a light circling pressure along the ridge of the skull with thumb or fingers.

9. Press in and up with your thumb at the depression just under the ridge of the skull. Work a line from near the ear into just beside the spine on one side, then the other. Your friend can take deep breaths as you hold. This is particularly good for headaches.

10. Gently slap the head with both hands, starting at the center of the top and working all around.

11. Let the slapping motion flow down onto the shoulders and change to a chopping motion with the sides of your hands, fingers loose (a more gentle massage) or straight. Ask your friend to lean forward and do the same chopping motion along the spinal muscles and back. Do it lightly also in the kidney area, just below the ribs.

12. Finish off by gently smoothing down the whole area you have massaged by slowly sliding your hands several times over your friend from the crown of the head to the tips of the shoulders.

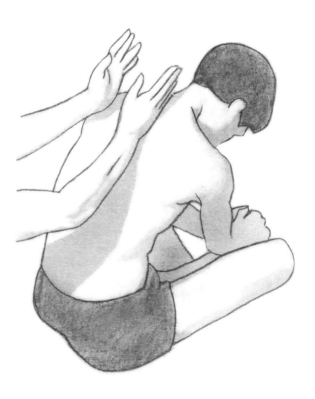

## The Principles

*Do-In* (pronounced "Doh-Een") is an ancient Oriental technique of self-massage that quickly relaxes and energizes the body by stimulating and harmonizing the flow of prana energy (in the East called *Chi* or *Ki*). It is based on the same principles as acupuncture, which works with the energy meridians (nerve channels that carry the energy of prana or *Chi* throughout the body) linking different organs. Thus, stimulating one point along a meridian will free the energy up and down the body along that channel.

In *Do-In*, when one part of the body is massaged, the less accessible parts, including inner organs, are also being stimulated. (Foot reflexology is based on the same principle.) *Do-In* is a wonderfully fast way to get your energy moving when you wake up in the morning, as well as to release tension at the end of the day.

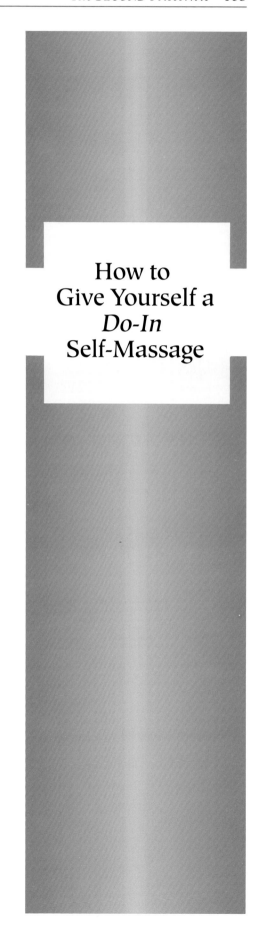

# How to Give Yourself a *Do-In* Self-Massage

## Step by Step Instructions

Take a comfortable position, preferably kneeling and sitting back on your heels. Relax and take some long, slow, deep breaths with your eyes closed and hands resting palms upward on your knees. When you feel calm and centered, you may begin.

Slowly stretch your arms up in the air above your head, extending your hands and fingers and tilting your head slightly back. Feel as if you are an empty cup, inviting the universal energy of prana to flow down into your being. Allow yourself to feel filled with energy before you start.

### 1. HEAD

Make loose fists with your hands and slowly bring them down to rest on the top of your head. Now begin gently to pound the top of your head, moving from the front to the back and from the center outward, and finishing with the back of the neck. That is good not only for the head, but also for the whole spine, the sinuses, and, at center top, for hemorrhoids.

### Ears

Gently pinch around the lobes of your ears with a rippling motion, starting at the top. Have your thumb on the front, fingers on the back. Then pinch and quickly pull your fingers away from three points: top, center, and lower lobe. That is beneficial for both the kidneys and the intestines. Rub up and down in front of your ears with your index finger until you feel heat. That is good for the small intestines.

### 2. FACE

### Forehead

Place your right hand in the palm of your left and bring both hands to rest lightly on your forehead. Keeping the hands still, gently turn your head from side to side so that it receives a gentle massage. Speed up slightly, then slow down again before stopping. That is very beneficial for the liver.

### Nose

Pinch the bridge of your nose firmly, hold for a few minutes, and then rub it. That is good for the sinuses and also the heart. Also pinch and massage your upper lip.

### Temples

Rub in a circular motion with three fingers to alleviate general tension.

### Eyes

With two fingers of each hand press gently all around the eyes, in a circle. Then cover them lightly with your palms for a short while and watch your inner sky.

### Cheeks

Vibrate them with your palms to stimulate the lungs. Then tap vigorously with fingertips all along the cheekbones, starting at the nose, and moving out and down in front of the ears to the angle of the jaw. That is good for large intestine, the sinuses, and also for depression.

### Jaw

With thumbs hooked under the jaw at its outside edge below the ear, and fingers on top, press in small circles toward the center. That helps relieve headaches and tension in the jaw and is good for the gums and teeth.

### Mouth

Tap vigorously with the fingertips, then massage, to benefit the gums and relieve tension. Stretch your mouth open and make noises. Move the jaw from side to side with your mouth wide open. That also facilitates release of tension.

Pause and shake out your hands. Feel as if you are shaking off tension and excess or static energy. Close your eyes for a moment and feel the prana circulating more freely in your head and face.

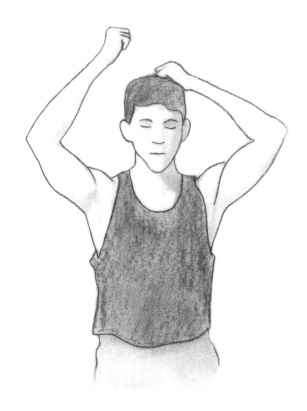

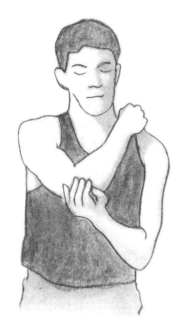

### 3. UPPER BODY

#### Neck and Shoulders

Make your right hand into a loose fist, bring it across your chest, and begin to pound vigorously down the left side of your neck and out to the tip of your shoulder. As you do that, support your right elbow in your left hand. Reach over to the back of your shoulder and pound the upper back muscle. It holds a great deal of tension. Reverse hands and do the same for your right neck and shoulder. That stimulates the eliminative process, particularly in the large intestine.

#### Arms

Again make your right hand into a fist and pound down the inside of your left arm (to stimulate the heart and lungs) and then up the outside (to stimulate the large and small intestines and to regulate body heat). Do that several times, then reverse arms.

#### Chest

Still with loose fists, pound the center of your upper chest at the start of your collarbone, moving out beneath it to your shoulders. Make a deep AAAHHH sound as you do so, to release tension and open up the lungs. That is particularly good if you have a cough. Then pound down the center of your upper body and out along the bottom edges of your rib cage. Be more gentle there, as you are working with your liver, spleen, and stomach.

#### Intestines

Gently pound your lower abdomen and pelvic area in clockwise circles (up the right side, across the top, and down the left) following the path of the colon.

Pause again to shake out your hands and to feel the energy moving in your body as you sit with eyes closed for a moment.

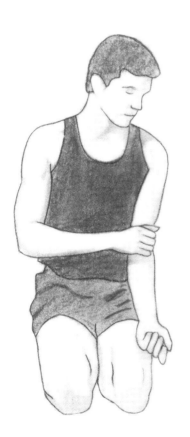

### 4. LEGS AND FEET

### Thighs

Pound vigorously down your thighs from pelvis to knee in three lines: center, inside, and outside. That is good for all your inner organs.

### Lower Back and Buttocks

Leaning forward, pound your lower back on either side of the spine down into the buttocks, ending at the small depressions. That is highly beneficial for the sciatic nerve and for the whole lower back. It is also good for the eliminative organs and for the kidneys (especially the higher areas).

### Legs

Stretch out your legs and gently thump them up and down on the floor, to release cramps and tension.

### Feet

First with one foot and then the other, repeat the following motions. Lift your foot up with both hands, knee bent, and shake it out. Rotate your foot around your ankle as you pinch the back of the ankle with the opposite hand to release any tension in the ankle joint. Place your foot, sole up, on your opposite thigh and begin to pound vigorously up and down on the sole.

Pounding on the sole stimulates your whole body, because the soles of the feet contain reflex points to the internal organs. Press your thumbs one on top of the other for strength, in four lines from the heel to the toes along the sole of the foot. One line will follow the inside edge of the foot, two will be in the middle and the fourth will be along the very outside edge. Rotate the toes one by one, starting with the big toe, then press each toe back toward the sole of the foot and out toward the front of the leg before snapping your fingers sharply off the end.

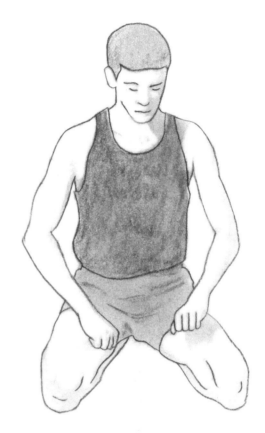

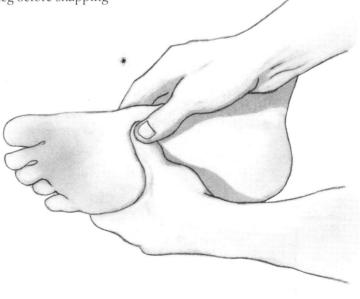

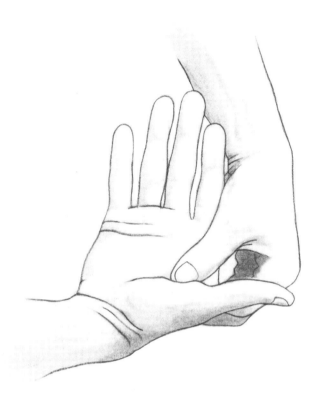

## 5. HANDS

Finally, massage your hands, which have just done all this hard work! First shake them out again to remove static energy and tiredness. Then, for each hand in turn, rotate and twist each finger with the whole of your other hand, bending it back and forth as you did with your toes. Crack your knuckles if you can, as that loosens the joints by redistributing the synovial fluid. Massage the palm of each hand with your fingers. This is good for the heart. Bite (gently!) the end of your little finger just to the outside of center near the top of the nail. That is also good for the heart and, reportedly, can even arrest a heart attack!

Massage the webbed area between your thumb and first finger. Find, by probing deeply, the tender spot there and massage it deeply. There are pressure points there for the sinuses and the intestines, and massaging that area will help headaches, constipation, and menstrual cramps. Shake out your hands one last time.

Sit quietly, with your eyes closed, and become sensitive to the energy that is moving more freely now in your body. Probably you feel quite different from the way you did before you started. Be aware of how you have refreshed and reenergized your whole body by this simple technique of self-massage. Promise yourself to stop and do it whenever you feel tension and tiredness in your body.

## STOP!

How aware are you of your body messages right now? How are you feeling? Is there tension, stiffness, or tiredness in any part of your body? Do you need to get up and stretch? Take some deep breaths? Relax your shoulders? Rest your eyes? Rest your mind? Close your eyes for a minute and take some long, slow, deep breaths to enable you to get in touch with your experience. Then respond to what your body is asking you to do.

# Other Health Tools

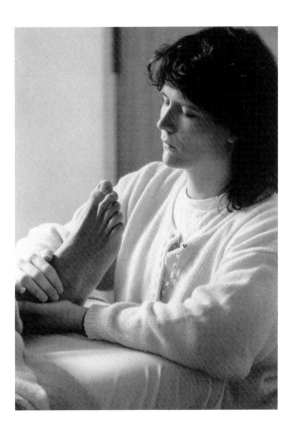

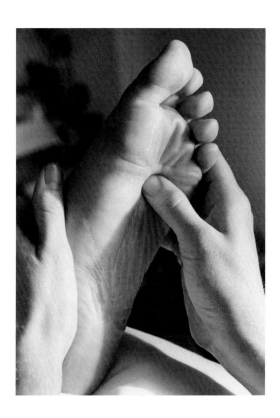

## Reflexology Foot Massage

Reflexology foot massage is an effective way to relax the whole body. All the energy currents throughout the body flow through the feet. The foot, by virtue of its accessibility, is easily massaged, and as the pressure points in the feet are stimulated the corresponding organs and areas of the body are balanced.

The potency of reflexology is based on the principle that every part of the body is reflexively connected to every other part. As the therapist locates and breaks up the crystalline salt deposits in the feet, the corresponding parts of the body are stimulated. That promotes the elimination of toxic wastes that have been produced through incomplete metabolism and stored in the tissues.

The musculature and fascia of the feet become supple and return to their original length and elasticity through massage. After experiencing this *kriya*, or yogic cleansing technique, many people say they feel a heightened sense of being grounded and supported as they stand and walk.

Reflexology is tremendously beneficial for those experiencing:

> constipation
> headache
> toothache
> tension
> backache
> shoulder pain
> indigestion
> overworked kidneys and gall bladder

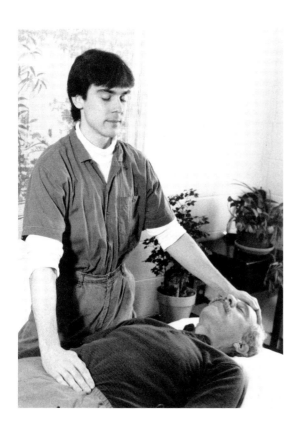

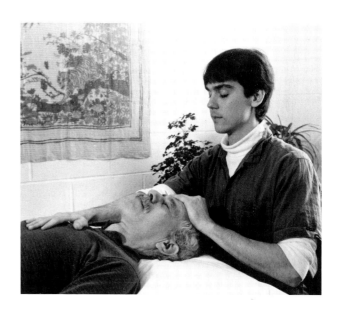

## Polarity Therapy

Polarity therapy is the science of balancing the vital life force in the body and is used to bring about deep, healing relaxation. When the energy poles in the body are restored to their equilibrium, a steady and peaceful feeling of health and well-being is experienced.

In a polarity session, gentle manipulations are used to direct the healing energy to specific areas in the body. The intelligent energy of the body is stimulated to break up physiological blocks and to restore the body's normal functioning.

The benefits of polarity are numerous, and extend to all persons, regardless of age or physical condition. They include

(1) structural realignment and reduction of muscular and skeletal pain;

(2) stimulation of all the vital organs and an energizing of the glandular system; and

(3) acceleration of the body's healing process promoted by the increase of available body energy.

# The Sauna

## The Sauna

A sauna, which not only relaxes the body but aids in its purification, uses dry heat to make the body perspire. Different methods for creating an environment to make the body sweat have been used for thousands of years, even before the times of the Greeks and Romans, to cleanse and relax the body. Cultures throughout the world, from Scandinavian to Native American, have used equivalents of the sauna as a tool for maintaining and enhancing health. The word *sauna* came to this country from Finland, where the sauna is an institution.

## What Happens to the Body During a Sauna?

A sauna uses heat to raise the temperature in the sauna room to 180 to 225 degrees Fahrenheit or more. Our bodies have a wonderful ability to adjust to such heat, primarily through the mechanism we call sweat. There are two million tiny sweat glands situated just below the surface of the skin. Each of those sweat glands is a tiny coiled tube that is connected to the blood circulation system and is capable of bringing water to the surface of the skin through tiny openings called pores.

When the temperature outside the body increases, the blood circulation within the body also increases as a means of distributing the heat throughout the body. You will notice during a sauna that your heart rate increases (sometimes up to 130 beats per minute, which is well above the norm of approximately seventy beats per minute).

When the temperature increases to a certain point, the sweat glands begin to secrete a liquid that is almost pure water, but also contains some undesirable mineral wastes from the body. Through the process of sweating and evaporation, the body is able to keep its inner temperature within a fairly constant range of 98 to 100 degrees Fahrenheit, even though the outside temperature is 180 degrees or more.

You might appreciate your body's wisdom even more if one day you mistakenly wore your watch into the sauna. You would soon find that the metal of your watch had become too hot to touch: metal doesn't sweat as our skin does. The process of bodily heat control is another example of the workings of prana, our body's innate intelligence that works automatically, without the intervention of our conscious mind, to preserve and enhance our health.

## What are the Benefits of a Sauna?

1. Relaxes the body and soothes the nerves: A sauna provides deep muscle relaxation for your body, as the increased circulation removes wastes from tired muscles and nerves, allowing them truly to relax and rest.

2. Cleanses and beautifies the body: In time, you'll have rosy skin as smooth as a baby's! All the pores of your body will open wide and your whole skin will be cleansed from inside out, as the top layer of dead skin cells will be sloughed off. The increased blood flow gives your skin a healthful vitality and look of aliveness.

3. Combats illness: During the fifteen to twenty minutes of a sauna, your body can dispose of waste elements that would otherwise take your kidneys over twenty-four hours to eliminate. Those accumulated waste elements in the body often lead to physical illness. The heat of a sauna helps eliminate those wastes and make you healthier in body, mind, and spirit.

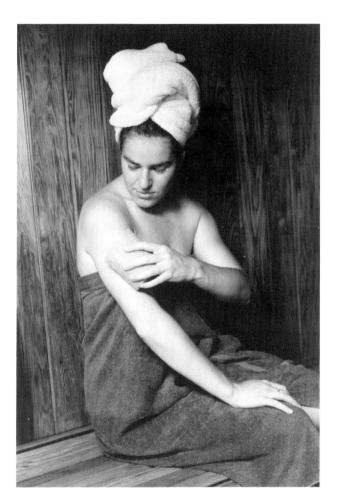

## How to Take a Sauna

The full sauna experience is a three-step process of
(1) heating up to a sweat in the sauna;
(2) cooling off rapidly in a cold shower; and
(3) returning to the sauna for relaxation.

Experienced sauna-goers may repeat that process three or four times in one sauna session. You will remember that the benefit of the sauna comes from increased blood circulation and sweating. The process of heating up and then cooling off rapidly tends to flush the inner organs with fresh blood, maximizing the benefits.

Sometimes people avoid the rapid cooling off because the cold water seems painful. That pain tends to disappear when you relax the body's muscles and breathe deeply in and out as the deliciously cool water stimulates the surface of your skin. For hours after, people often feel a warm glow of heat that seems to come from deep within the body: another experience of prana.

A common sauna practice is to rub the surface of the skin before and during the sauna with a loofa, which is a dried gourd sponge that stimulates the blood circulation when rubbed on the skin. A dry, natural-bristle brush is also very effective.

Be sure that you are gentle with yourself in your first sauna experience. Don't allow yourself to become dizzy with too much heat exposure. Most people find that five to ten minutes is enough time in the sauna at first. Each person is different, so judge your own capacity. You may want to begin your first sauna by sitting on the lower bench where the temperature tends to be lower.

## Who Should Not Take a Sauna

Anyone with medical problems, particularly those related to the heart or circulatory system, including hypertension and high or low blood pressure, should consult a doctor before taking a sauna, as it may not be advisable.

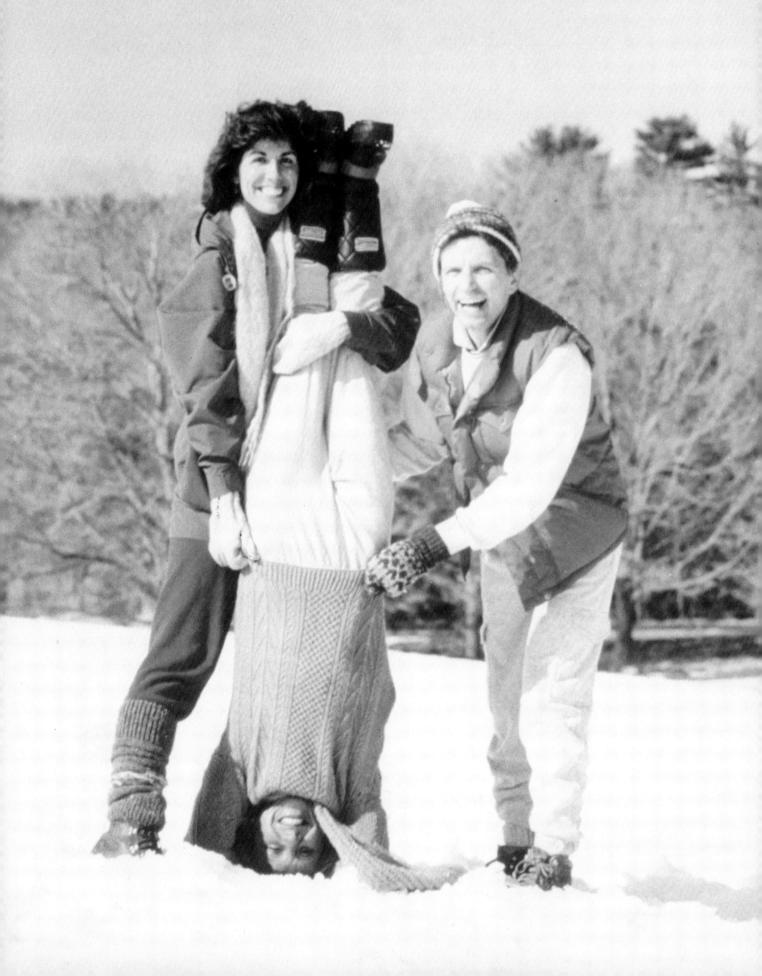

# The Third Pathway

## learning how to play

# Can You Come out to Play?

The steps to holistic health that have been discussed so far are probably no surprise to you, but where does learning to play fit in? Play has become something that mature adults are not expected to do or take seriously. Sports, cultural activities, creative arts, studying — those are praiseworthy and acceptable ways to spend the time when we are not working. But playing? Adults don't play, do they?

That is the whole problem. We seem to have accepted the idea that any activity that has no goal (such as defeating an opponent) or tangible end result (such as winning a trophy) and does not demand concentration and brain power (such as chess or bridge) is not a valid way to spend time. We play with our children occasionally, but with each other? Hardly.

Yet play (light-hearted activity that has no apparent purpose) is an essential ingredient in holistic health, as are laughter and humor. If we enter fully into play, we lose ourselves in the fun of it and our minds and bodies relax as they become united in the activity. Laughter is deeply relaxing because it loosens up the abdomen, releasing stress from the solar plexus where tension is stored.

Most of us take our lives far too seriously. If we could learn to laugh a little at our problems, to see the humor inherent in almost any situation, we would be more relaxed and healthier people. There is a child within each of us who longs to be let out to play. Learning how to contact and enjoy that childlike aspect of ourselves is a vital part of the Kripalu Approach to holistic health.

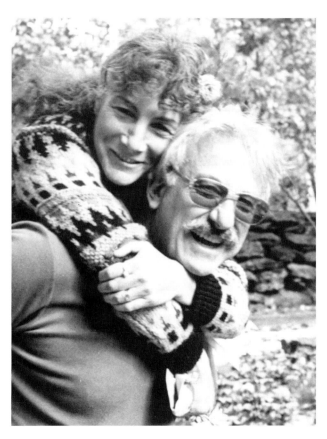

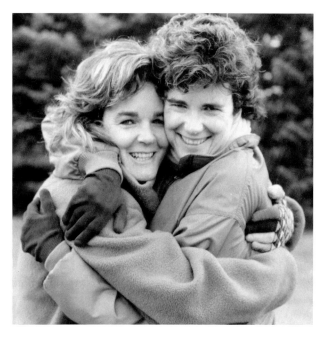

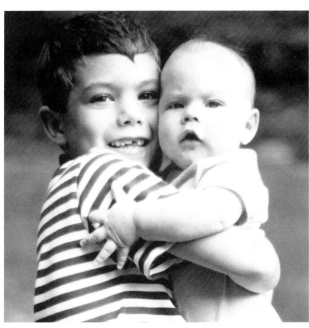

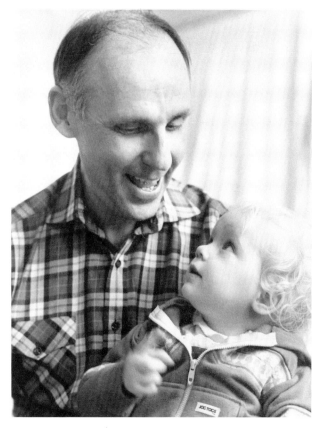

# The Healing Power of Laughter, Play, and Humor

"Good spirits are a vital part of life. Denying joy is one of the greatest deprivations on this planet!" So remarked Norman Cousins, long-time Editor of Saturday Review and guest lecturer at UCLA Medical School. What was a journalist doing at a medical school? Teaching people how to heal with humor!

Cousins' expertise came from direct experience. In 1964, he developed a serious collagen illness that weakened the connective tissues of his body and was said to be a degenerative condition. Since his body reacted to almost all the medication given him in the hospital, Cousins began to search for alternatives.

He had read Dr. Hans Selye's *The Stress of Life* and began to question whether his emotions played a hand in his illness. If so, could it be possible that positive emotions could create positive chemical changes in the body as well? As he said, "Is it possible that love, hope, laughter, and the will to live have a therapeutic value?"

Cousins decided to test that hypothesis. In partnership with his physician, Dr. William Hitzig, he began a regimen that included using laughter as a healing force along with activities designed to affirm positive emotions. It worked. Watching classics from the TV show "Candid Camera" was particularly effective.

"I made the joyous discovery that ten minutes of genuine belly laughter had an anesthetic effect and would give me at least two hours of pain-free sleep." As time passed and he continued his therapy, the connective tissue in his body began to regenerate. In subsequent years he resumed jogging and horseback riding and was almost pain free.

In summarizing what he learned, Cousins said, "Never underestimate the capacity of the human mind and body to regenerate — even when the prospects seem wretched. The life-force may be the least-understood force on earth. William James said that human beings tend to live too far within self-imposed limits. It is possible that those limits will recede when we respect more fully the natural drive of the human mind and body toward perfectibility and regeneration. Protecting and cherishing that natural drive may well represent the finest exercise of human freedom."*

How did the healing of Norman Cousins happen? Consider, for a moment, the last time you had a hearty belly laugh or played a relaxed game of golf or sandlot baseball, or got together with a group of friends for an evening game of Monopoly or Pictionary! Where was your mind at the time? How did you feel emotionally? What was the experience of your body?

---

*Quotations and story from *New England Journal of Medicine*, December, 1976.

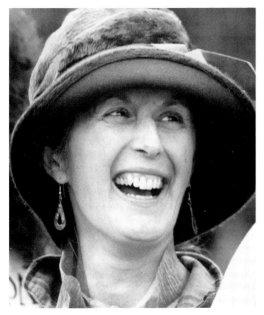

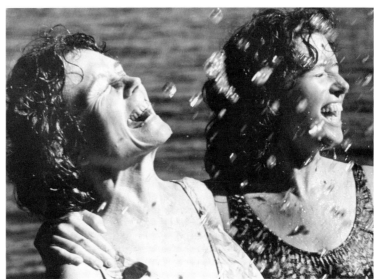

## Laughter and Prana

If you consult your experience, you'll most likely agree that play and humor are indeed captivating. And what do they capture us from? They save us from our reveries (and regrets) about the past and our hopes and anxieties about the future. Play and humor bring our minds into the moment. We become concentrated, without effort. We become absorbed, without tension.

Through play and humor, prana, the inner life force that Cousins called "the least understood . . . on earth," is freed to manifest and flow within us. When we play and laugh, our prana is in harmony with the world and the people around us. Free of roles, conflicting attitudes, and social dictums, our bodies and minds relax into the energy of life. Energy is ignited rather than spent, creating an explosion of good feelings, positivity, and connectedness.

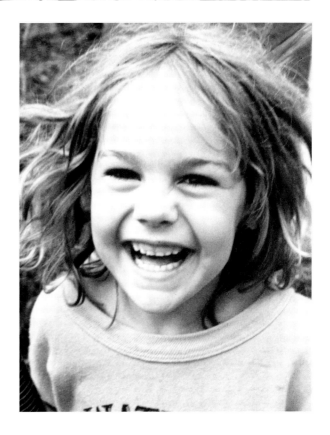

Earlier, disease was defined as a condition wherein the flow of prana has been blocked and chronically denied expression. In the experience of play or humor, we enter a world of ease, effortless freedom, and faith. Mind, body, and prana are harmonized. In this act of letting go, prana is freed to do the work of healing.

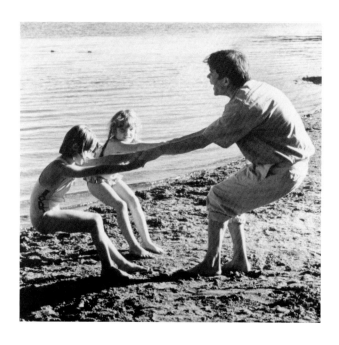

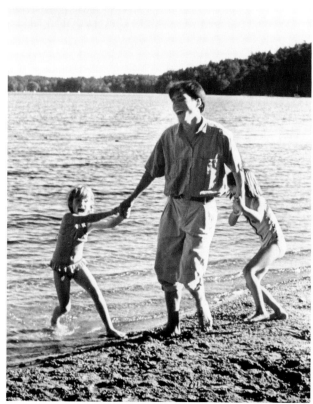

# The Child Within

No one has to teach children how to play or laugh. For them everything is new; therefore, they are delighted at the simplest things. Can you imagine a child thinking: "Gee, I haven't taken time to play this week; maybe I should plan an hour to have some fun?" At the same time, have you ever known an adult who forgot to eat, even once a day? So we all have priorities in life, some conscious and some unconscious, and they have a tremendous influence on us.

Because of our priorities, many of us have lost some of the innocent qualities we possessed as children. We've become so caught up in the ambitious endeavor of making our dreams come true that we're too busy to play anymore, so we miss the joy and fun that brought us such pleasure.

Children make fun out of everything they do. A few pebbles can become a castle; a little breeze and a kite have endless possibilities! As grown-ups, our ability to enjoy life through play has become covered up by the pressures and attitudes of our concept of grown-up life. Yet all we need do to reactivate that ability is to rediscover the child within us.

A child lives close to prana, that is, close to inner needs and natural responses uncensored by the mind. That same dynamic is experienced when we laugh and play. That is why we feel like kids when we're experiencing ourselves in that way.

Much has been written in the past decade about reconnecting with and nurturing the child within us. Psychology has asserted that we become adult too soon and remain in that role too much, mistakenly thinking that our well-being will flourish if we are mature and remain in control.

The child lets go of life. In the act of playing, our bodies once again move naturally and effortlessly; in the act of laughing, our hearts open to the joy that is inherent in each of us.

We need to rediscover the child within us and nurture it as another step on the path to holistic health. The following exercises have been designed to help you do just that.

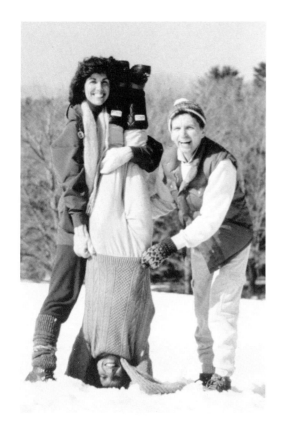

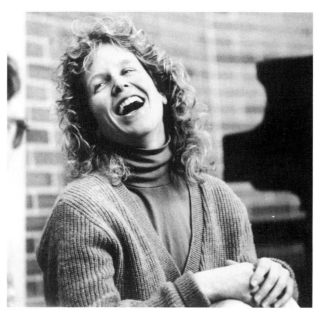

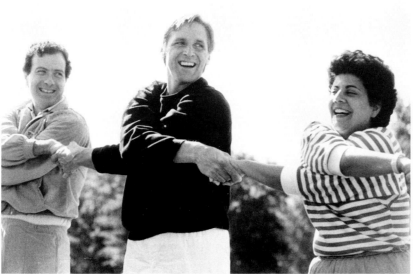

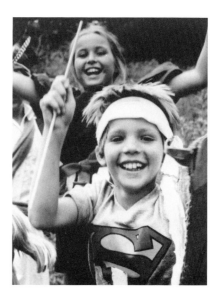

# Self-Discovery Experience 10

## Getting to know the playful child within you

This experience is a little different from previous ones. You will need

1. some sheets of sketching paper;
2. lined notebook paper;
3. if possible, some colored crayons or pencils; and
4. a mirror.

## Awareness

1. Sit very still and see if you can remember something recent or from some time ago that gave you a really good belly laugh. Allow yourself to remember it so vividly (it may help to close your eyes) that you begin to laugh heartily again at the memory. It may take some time, but just relax until you recapture the memory and the feeling. If you are unable actually to reexperience the laughter, simply try to recall how your body felt when you laughed. Now, at this moment how do you feel, physically, emotionally, and mentally? Write it down.

2. If you weren't able to get in touch with your laughter, how does that make you feel right now? How do you respond when other people are laughing and you don't find it funny? Write those thoughts down.

3. Reflect for a moment. How often do you really laugh? Is it often enough for you? Do you sometimes wish you were able to laugh more? Do you wish that more funny/laughable things happened in your life? How do you feel about laughter, humor, play, and the role they have in your life right now? Write those feelings down also.

4. After reading the instructions, close your eyes and go through the following visualization: See yourself as a very small child, laughing and playing with other children. Try to feel how it felt to be that child. See how he or she was playing, and feel the emotions and bodily sensations.

   When you've really immersed yourself in the experience, open your eyes and without thinking start to draw or sketch the images that come to you to express what you experienced in the visualization. It is important to drop any old tapes that say, "I can't draw" or "I'm not artistic." Just transfer your images to paper, knowing that no one will see them but you. They may be drawings that depict you as a child, with the toys and games you played, or they may be abstract shapes and images that symbolize the feelings. You can write in single words, too, if they seem to fit.

5. Close your eyes again and repeat the visualization process with a later stage in your childhood — maybe at age eight or nine. Again, without thinking, draw the images that come to you as you open your eyes. Thinking often becomes judging and can stifle the innate creativity brought to the surface by prana.

   Repeat the process three more times: for your teenage years, your young adulthood, and the present moment.

6. Review all your sketches and notes and see what they tell you about yourself, your attitudes to play and humor, and how you have changed over the years. What did you laugh at then and now? How fully did you/do you laugh and how often? Write down your observations.

7. Try to see any patterns that are preventing you from being more playful and humorous in the present. Do you have an inner parent telling you something like "grow up," "be sensible," "stop being childish," "don't be lazy," "don't be silly," or "act your age"? Do you have old tapes in your head, containing messages that say "playing is just for children," "mature adults don't play," or "if you want to be respected and taken seriously you can't afford to fool around or be lighthearted"? (Those are just some samples; your own tapes may be different).

8. Do you really believe that play and humor are important parts of life and contributors to health? Did you in the past?

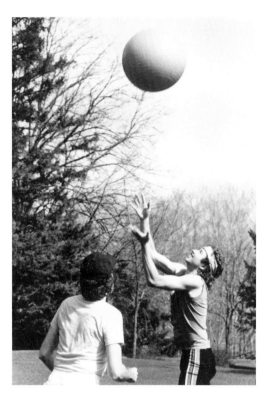

## Acceptance

9. Sitting quietly, absorb what you have learned about yourself and make it part of you. Feel good about it, as if that part of you were a new friend you had just made. Feel what it means to you — how it changes the image you have held of yourself — and be glad you can now adjust to a more accurate and enjoyable self-concept.

10. Make a drawing of your inner child.

11. Speak to that newly discovered child who has been hiding inside just waiting to be allowed out to play. As if you were the loving, nurturing parent of this child, ask him or her: "What do you need from me? What would you like me to do so that you may express yourself through play and humor?" Listen to the response of the prana-child and write it down.

12. Now look at yourself in the mirror and smile!

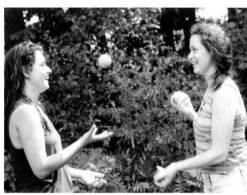

## Adjustment

13. Start writing down all the ways in which you can safely express your inner child and meet its needs. Be specific as to what you will do, when, with whom, and how often.

14. Gather ideas from the following "How to" section to incorporate into your new play scheme.

15. Resolve to nurture your inner child consciously, saying when you are pleased with him or her, encouraging him or her to be daring and fearless, and lovingly supporting his or her emergence and growth, just as you would that of a real child — for it is a real child. It is the child you once were, who had to grow up too soon or became afraid to express and enjoy itself because adults disapproved of its high spirits (only because the children in them had unknowingly been squashed by their parents and teachers; the chain of cause and effect recedes into infinity).

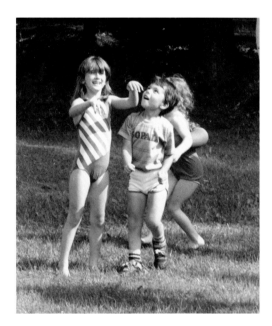

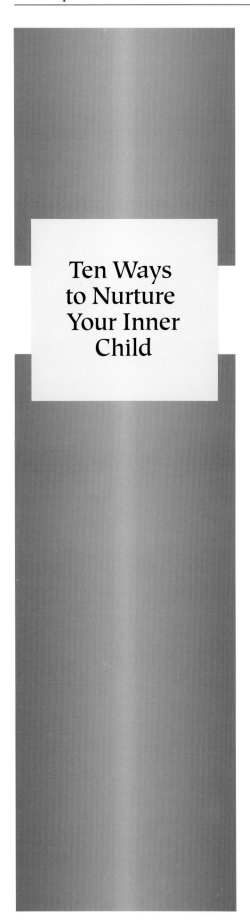

## Ten Ways to Nurture Your Inner Child

1. Be with children and play with them or at least observe them play. See their total absorption in what they are doing, how lost they are in it. See how freely they laugh at the smallest things, not caring what the laughter sounds or looks like. Notice their complete lack of inhibition and self-criticism.

2. Laugh for the pure pleasure of laughing, not because something is funny and you are laughing at it. You may have to force yourself at first and you may feel phony or be embarrassed by the sound of your own laughter. In actual fact, your forced laughter is more real than your habitual seriousness, for laughter is innate in all of us. We have simply lost the spontaneity of it. Deep, full laughter involves muscles that may not have been used for a long time and so may need practice — a kind of remedial exercise!

3. Find yourself a buddy to have fun with and practice on each other! Pick someone you trust fully and have no fear of being judged or rejected by, otherwise you won't be able to express yourself fully.

4. Laugh, don't just smile! Will Durant said, "The smile is sometimes an abortion of a laugh."

5. Laugh at yourself. Cultivate a more detached attitude toward the situations you consider to be problems or difficulties, so that you can see the humor inherent in them. Life is not so serious really. Sincerity is one thing, seriousness another.

6. Look at the world through a child's eyes — empty, wondering, marvelling at the ever-new panorama unfolding before you.

7. Do something playful, different, and spontaneous every day. Be careful, though, to choose appropriate people and places. Someone who has not reawakened the inner child may not see the joke.

8. Read children's books for their freshness and humor. We especially like *Winnie-the-Pooh* by A.A. Milne and *The Secret Garden* by Frances Hodgson Burnett.

9. Share your joy. "A sorrow that's shared is but half the trouble, but a joy that's shared is a joy made double."

10. Play games with yourself and others. Here's a list to help you get started:

1. **Card and board games:** old favorites like *Monopoly* and *Scrabble* and newer games like *Feeling Good* and *Pictionary.*

2. **Charades.** (When was the last time you played and really enjoyed it?)

3. **Kids' races** using wheelbarrows, sacks, or eggs and spoons.

4. **Dress-up games.** (Remember how as a kid you loved to dress up?)

5. **Crazy team games.** For example:

   (a) Each member has to do something like dress up in old clothes of the opposite sex and race to a point and back.

   (b) Each team has five minutes to form itself into an animal; then it parades in front of the other team(s) who have to guess its identity.

   (c) Two teams face each other. A member of one team starts at one end of the two rows and a member of the other starts at the opposite end. As they walk between the teams, passing each other in the middle, they must not laugh. The other members of each team are supposed to do everything in their power (short of physical contact) to make their opponents' member laugh or smile. A loser goes to the other team.

   (d) Tug-of-War.

   Those are just examples, of course. Have the fun of making up your own.

6. **"Experience" games.** One such game is done in groups of three or four. One person must become totally slack and relaxed; the others are to gently lower that person to the ground, then lift them up to a standing position again. (You won't believe how heavy a totally relaxed body is. Sometimes three other people cannot lift the person.) Then have someone tense up his or her whole body like a board, and see how easy he or she is to lift.

7. **Fun by yourself.**

   (a) When no one is around, put on some dance music and dance all by yourself. Do it to wear yourself out, to express all your energy, like a high-spirited child.

   (b) Run rather than walk sometimes, not like a jogger but like a free child. Skip and jump, leap into puddles, go barefoot, eat with your fingers, sing songs to yourself — in short, be a child for a while.

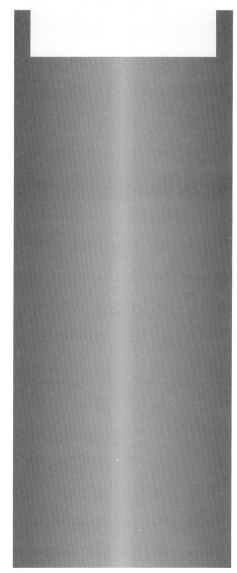

# Games to Play Just for the Fun of It

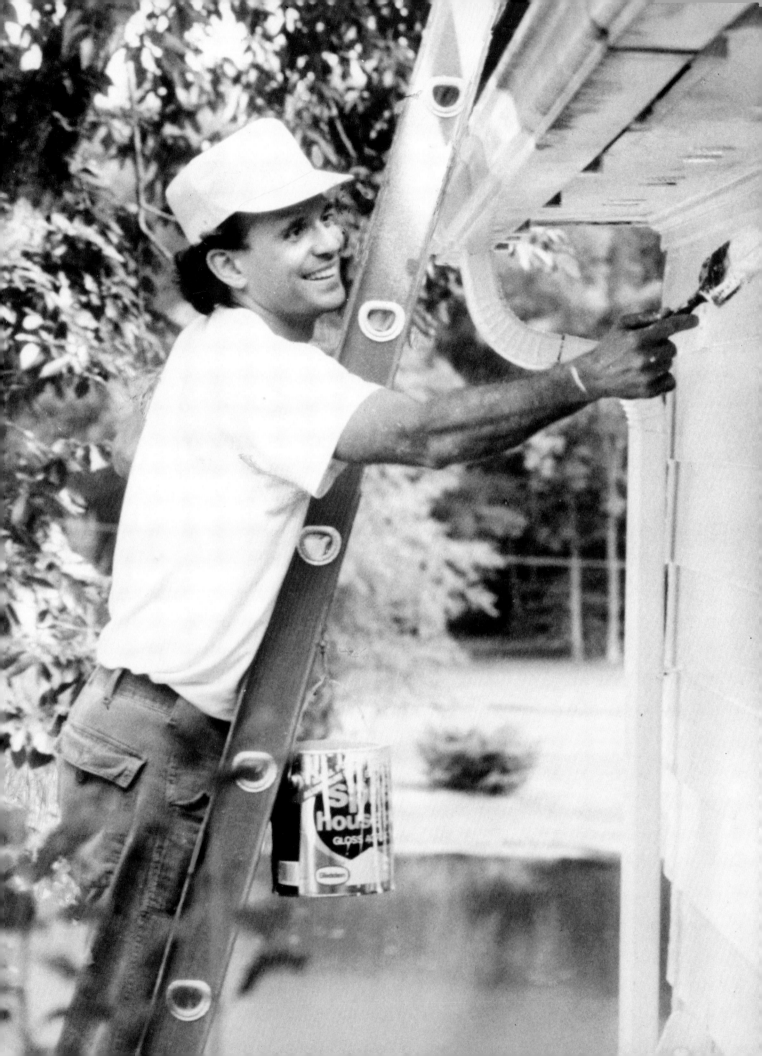

# *The Fourth Pathway*

## learning the art of relaxed work

# Work:
# Expressing Our Creative Energy

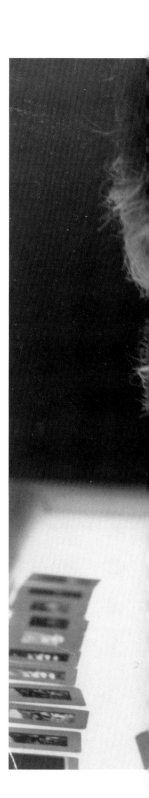

Eight hours a day, five days a week, fifty weeks a year — from the time we learn to make our own bed until the time we plant our post-retirement garden — in all those hours of all those years, we are doers. Work is an expression of our energy, our bodies, our minds, our hearts, our souls, our creative potential. It is no wonder it deserves our attention as a pathway to the experience of happiness and well-being.

The articles and exercises that follow give you opportunities to explore the place that work holds in your approach to life and health and to develop ways in which it might make an even greater contribution to your well-being and happiness.

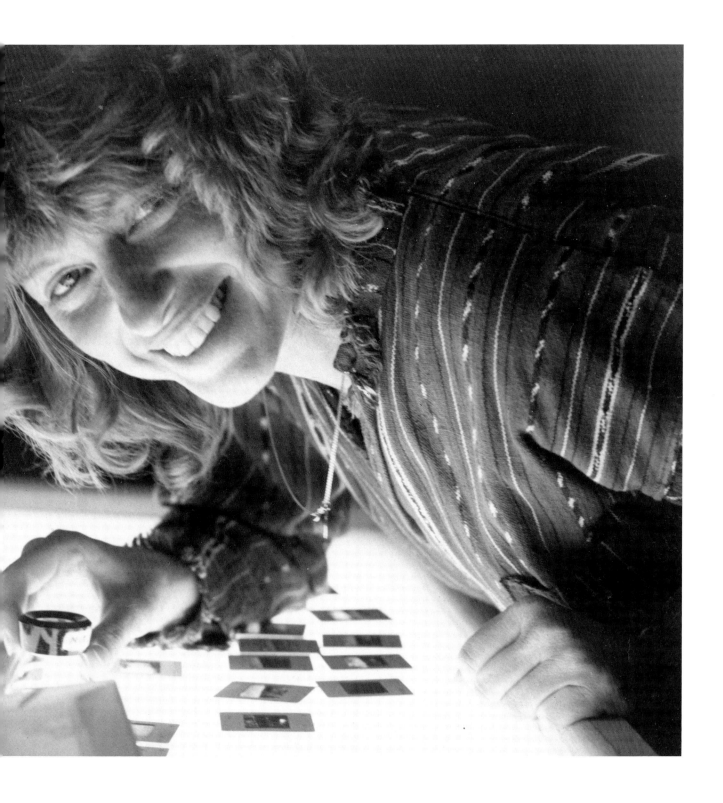

## Work and Relaxation — Opposites?

The very word *work* conjures up the opposite of relaxation for many people. However much we may like our jobs, work means effort. Relaxation is something we do on weekends or on vacation (in other words, when we're not working). Yet work and relaxation need not be separate. That is a fundamental part of the Kripalu Approach to holistic health and its cornerstone of free-flowing prana energy.

As we have already seen, the key to free-flowing prana is relaxation in everything we do, including work. But how can we be relaxed at work? Some people just are; some jobs seem to preclude it. Loving what you do helps, but even then stress can creep in. Isn't it inevitable that we should feel tired by five o'clock every afternoon and exhausted by Friday? After all, working hard for forty hours a week or so is tiring, isn't it? Not necessarily.

Yogi Desai, for instance, puts in more hours a week than almost anyone we know in a normal job. He directs Kripalu Center, counsels and provides spiritual guidance to many, teaches workshops and seminars across this country and around the world, yet never seems to be tired. His energy seems to be boundless. What is his secret?

The secret is conservation of energy, which means two things: (1) spending the energy we have cautiously and wisely, that is, not wasting or draining it or letting it leak away unconsciously, and (2) learning to draw in more than the average amount of energy.

There are two main areas to work on in energy conservation, then. First, we must learn to be more aware of what is happening to the energy in our bodies and examine and change stress-causing attitudes (as we found in the previous chapter). In this chapter we will explore attitudes about work that may cause us to experience it as tiring and tension producing.

Second, it is helpful to learn to draw more energy into the body. That is explained in more detail in The Seventh Pathway, in an article entitled "The Meditation of Natural Living."

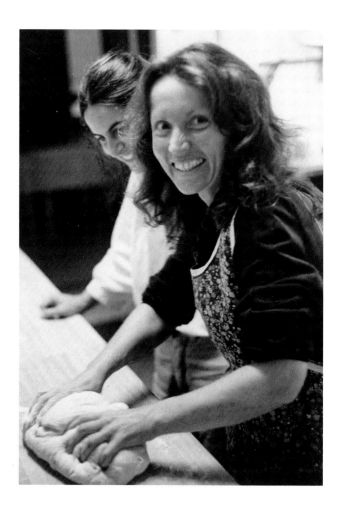

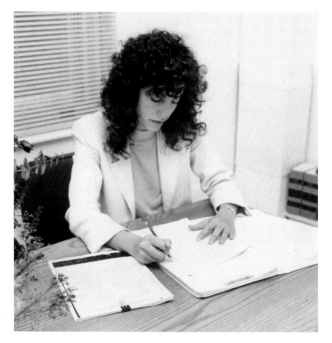

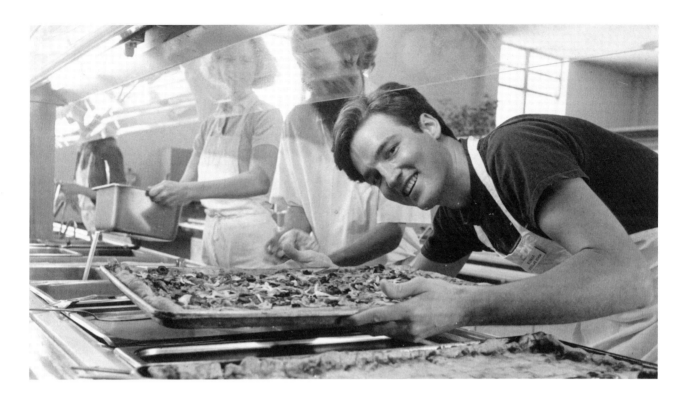

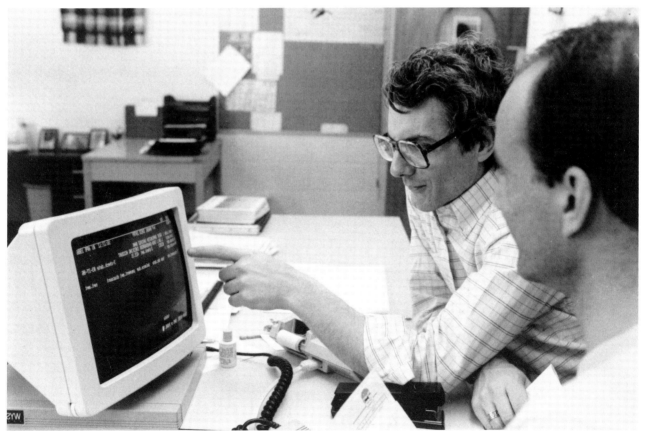

# Self-Discovery Experience

# 11

## What do your hidden attitudes about work reveal to you?

### DIRECTIONS:

Get paper and pencil and set aside thirty quiet minutes alone to do this introspection.

## Awareness

1. Take an inventory of your perceptions about and definitions of work. Close your eyes, relax, and let your mind dwell on what work means to you. Then, on a piece of paper, list and/or draw the words, phrases, and images you associate with the activity called work. Put down whatever comes, without evaluating or criticizing it.

2. See yourself going through a typical work day. Start from the beginning, perhaps as you get out of bed, preparing yourself to go to work. Come in touch with the feelings about work that you experience in each phase of the day. List or draw those feelings and the ways they find expression. For example: "frustrated driving to work, so I blew my horn in traffic jam" or "excited about new project, so I am enthusiastic in talk with Jim."

3. Now complete the following statement, being as honest with yourself as you can: "I work because . . . " List everything that comes to mind, both the practical reasons and the more subtle.

4. Finally, list honestly whom it is important for you to please through your work. After each name, list what it is you hope to receive from that person as a result of your work.

5. If you have more than one kind of work (e.g., a housewife who also holds an outside job), explore the differences in attitude you have about your various jobs.

## Acceptance

6.   Reread your responses to number 1. For each, write down what or who it was that influenced that definition or perception about work. Take stock of which perceptions still appear reasonable when you look at them consciously and objectively.

7.   Consider numbers 3, 4, and 5. Look over each list and write down what your true, underlying needs may be. For example, you may have said that you want your boss to give you a pat on the back, but what you are really needing is to feel accepted.

8.   Consider numbers 4 and 5 once again. Close your eyes and see clearly the persons you listed. Going beyond your formal relationship with them (your role and theirs), be with the person behind the title or role. Come in touch with what you sincerely desire to feel between the two of you and write it down.

9.   Consider number 2 above. Complete the statement: "I express my feelings about my work in this way rather than in another because . . . " Reflect on ways of increasing your awareness of how your feelings influence your behavior and attitudes at work.

10.   Reread all your answers and see to what extent you have a pattern of identifying yourself as what you do and basing your self-esteem on that, rather than simply on who you are.

## Adjustment

After doing the above exercises, you should have a clearer picture of your attitudes and feelings about your work. Reread all that you have recorded to get an overview of who you are as a doer. Are there any inconsistencies, needs, or perceptions that appear as patterns in each response?

You may find, for example, a consistent perception that "I should always work hard or others won't value me." Once you have seen that, you can then consider whether or not it is true. If you reflect on all your findings in that way, you will discover a whole repertoire of actions you can take to make your work more pleasurable and a fuller expression of who you really are.

Sitting quietly, let the actions you'd like to take to make your work more effective and bring you more happiness emerge as a knowing from your intuition. Write those actions down. They may include some of the following:

11.   A redefinition of what work means to you, now. Decide on a definition that you feel is healthy and reasonable and that you want to live with, and let it direct your actions and attitudes as you work.

12.   Some simple, specific ways to reduce tension and conflict. Focus on any pattern of feelings about work that express tension or conflict and decide on new ways you can approach the situation. Beginning with the physical is usually the easiest. For example, choose to do deep breathing during a traffic jam. After relaxing, you may get in touch with the real reason for your tension; if it is because you need to talk with your boss about giving you fifteen minutes leeway in arriving in the morning, you may now be calm and trusting enough to do so.

13.   Some ways to share your needs and fears with others. After getting clear about what it is you really would like to receive from the significant people in your life, consider ways to share your needs with them. Your honesty may result in their being able to be more open with you. You will then know what their needs are and how those needs can also be met through a more open communication or relationship.

14.   A change in your own attitudes. You may discover that the simplest and yet most powerful way to change your experience of work is to change the way you perceive it.

# Freeing Yourself from Work

## Looking at Your Expectations

In the final analysis, it is our concepts and attitudes about work that decide how much pleasure and fulfillment we get. In addition to relaxing physically at work, we need to cultivate an attitude of relaxation toward the work we do. That does not mean becoming passive and never trying to get ahead or improving efficiency or having a career. It simply means checking out our underlying attitudes, seeing where they cause us tension, and relaxing them.

The most common tension-producing attitude, and perhaps the one we are least aware of, is expectation. Without realizing it, we may expect to get our work done in a certain amount of time, with the complete cooperation of external circumstances, including other people. Or, depending on the underlying attitudes we hold, we may expect nothing to go right.

So we anticipate praise or blame; a promotion or criticism; whatever it is, good or bad, we are always unconsciously expecting something. And that creates permanent tension in us. The first step in learning to enjoy our work more is to drop, or at least become more aware of, our expectations and simply become absorbed in the moment-to-moment completion of each task in the best possible way.

## Focusing on the Process Rather than the Results

The second most common cause of tension is being result oriented. We have to care, of course, about the results of our labor and put forth our best effort — nothing less is worthy of us as conscious beings. Yet we often tend to focus so much of our energy and attention on the final result that we cannot enjoy the process.

If we think all the time of how nice it will be when a particular task is finished, or are anxious about the result, we take ourselves out of the present and lose the pleasure of that moment. Relaxation can only truly come when we are in the experience of the moment, not the thought of the future.

In the West we tend to be excessively time conscious. If we observe ourselves as we go about our daily tasks, we will probably catch ourselves with many thoughts of "How quickly can I get this task done and move on?" We constantly pressure ourselves about time, all the while imagining that it is the job, the boss, the client, or the family that are demanding too much from us.

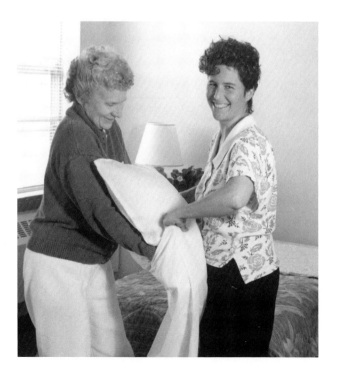

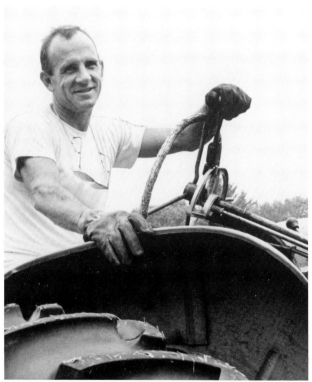

## Realigning Your Values

This time consciousness is related to a value consciousness that is also tension producing: "This task is more important (or interesting or valuable or worth my time) than that one." "This job is not as rewarding as his/hers." "If only I had a more fulfilling job, I'd be happy."

Some jobs are intrinsically more interesting than others, but our attitude toward the job is the most important ingredient. Without the right attitude, no job, however fascinating, will ever satisfy us, because every job has its downside: the chores, the repetition, or perhaps the dangers and tensions.

Our inappropriate value system comes from identifying ourselves with what we do. "Who are you?" "I am an executive." "I am a housewife." "I am a student." We need to remember we are not what we do. What we do as an occupation is simply one of many expressions of our energy. That pattern started very early in life: Even in grade school, we felt good about ourselves if we got an "A" and bad if we got a "C" or "D."

Our need to do, to succeed, and to accomplish is often an expression of our deep human need to feel accepted. Unfortunately, if we work with an unconscious motivation of gaining love and acceptance through our job, we will always experience the tension of the underlying fear of not getting that acceptance.

That is one source of tension that seems to be the hardest for us to see objectively. It runs like a thread through all the others. Unconsciously we are always asking, "What an I getting out of this?" "Am I being paid enough?" "Am I getting the respect/gratitude that I deserve?" That viewpoint is unproductive because it generates tension.

Actually, we can seldom be sure that we are getting what we feel is due us. At moments of success, such as receiving a promotion or a pay increase or special praise, it may feel that way, but those times are infrequent. So tension will underlie our work whenever we are looking at it only in terms of gain. If we can focus instead on the ways that our work is a service to others and a giving rather than a getting, we will automatically become more relaxed.

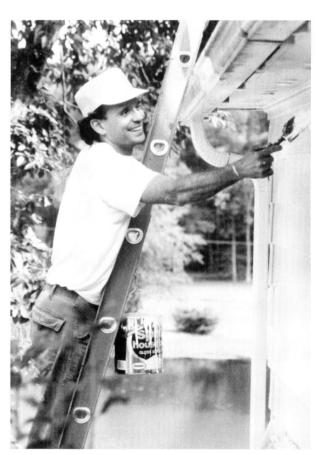

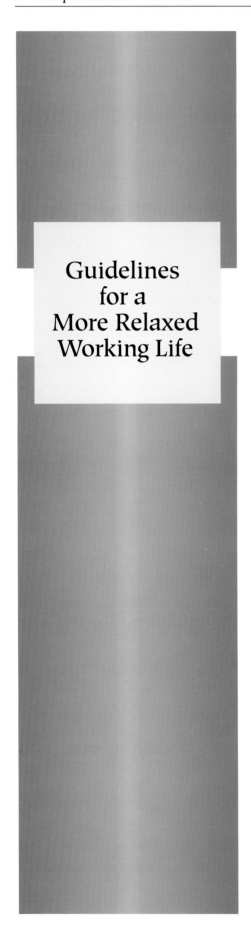

## Guidelines for a More Relaxed Working Life

1. Remain physically relaxed by stopping to do stretching or deep breathing throughout the day. Get plenty of exercise and fresh air and make every movement of your body flowing and harmonious, conserving as much energy as possible.

2. Observe your tensions, and use them as messages from which you can learn about yourself.

3. Become conscious of your expectations. If you see them clearly, they won't prevent you from fully accepting and enjoying what is actually happening.

4. Focus more on the moment-to-moment process of what you are doing and less on the end result, which will take care of itself if you are fully efficient in each moment.

5. Let time be your friend, not a constant opponent with which you must fight. Get lost in the moment: lift the pressure of self-imposed deadlines and plan realistically, then just do your best in each moment and you'll be able to drop anxiety.

6. Concentrate on drawing your self-esteem and sense of identity from all that you are as a unique individual, rather than from what you do. See what you do as simply a partial expression of your energy.

7. See all tasks as of equal value in terms of your growth as a whole person. How well you do something, and with what care and attention, is of more importance and value than the mere label attached to the task.

8. Begin to look at your work in terms of how it can help others. As you do something routine, imagine the satisfaction and pleasure someone will ultimately receive from your wholehearted, giving action. For instance, if you are folding laundry, really feel how much pleasure the person will receive as they see and smell the neatly folded laundry. Or if you're writing a memo, imagine how well-informed and helped the recipient is going to feel, even if you never hear it from them.

See your work as service, in the highest sense of the word, to others and to yourself. By helping others to the best of your ability, you are helping yourself to grow into a happier, freer, more relaxed, and fully alive human being. And that is what we all want.

The effects of these changes of attitude toward your work will be profound. You will find yourself being more relaxed, flowing through your day without getting ruffled by things that used to bother you. You will be less tired at the end of the day, with more energy to do activities you've wanted to find time for. And you will feel in tune with your prana and be more and more in the moment, so that time passes unnoticed and boredom and tension become things of the past.

# APPLYING THE PRINCIPLES
# OF KARMA YOGA TO YOUR WORK
### by Yogi Amrit Desai

**K**arma Yoga is an attitude rather than an action. It is an important attitude, toward work and life, which is well worth cultivating if we wish to achieve holistic health, because it will enable us to experience complete freedom from tension. That is the state in which our prana flows freely and our mind, body, and spirit are functioning in perfect harmony.

## Dropping Anxiety About Results

What is the attitude of Karma Yoga? It is carrying out our daily tasks and responsibilities, whether at home or work, in a spirit of equanimity, without anxiety about the results of our actions. It means cultivating a calm and accepting attitude, no matter what happens. It means being dispassionate about the end result, that is, dropping any fear of failure, desire for success, or wanting things to happen in a certain way.

If we worry about results, our passions and emotions are constantly involved in what is happening. As a result, we are always carrying tension with us. Westerners have become very result oriented and that is why the level of tension in this society is so high. Many people base their whole lives on achieving their concept of success or on meeting specific goals within a specific time frame.

It is not wrong to have a sense of direction and commitment. On the contrary, those are very important aspects of life. But there is a big difference between a goal and a direction, between commitment and attachment. Goals and attachments bring us tension and suffering; direction and commitment bring self-knowledge and inner peace.

## Seeing Work as Service

Given the conditions of their lives and occupations in our tense society, many people find it impossible to believe that they can attain to such a level of equanimity and calm acceptance of whatever happens. Yet it is really not so difficult once we understand the concept. It takes only time, practice, patience — and a new attitude: that of selfless service.

Karma Yoga looks at the activities of work in terms of helping others, rather than furthering one's success and reputation. When we are able to drop our egotistical motives, we dissolve our work tensions because we no longer have any anxiety about results. We can then work with relaxation and equanimity, gaining satisfaction from helping others.

Our life was given us to help others, not simply ourselves. Giving and receiving is a law of nature, and whenever we experience unhappiness in life, it is because we have gone against that law and tried to receive more than we gave. Unhappiness is nature's way of reminding us that we must participate in the universal law of giving and receiving.

We feel good about ourselves when we give to others and help them; we feel bad when we ignore the needs of others and step over them to achieve our own ends. Most of our unhappiness and self-rejection comes from an inner awareness that we may not consciously recognize: we are subtly aware that we are always wanting something for ourselves and, therefore, are seldom able to perform any action that is truly selfless.

## Dropping the Achievement Syndrome

Everyone wants to be happy. We believe that what will make us happy is the approval, acceptance, and love of others. We also believe that to get that approval and acceptance we must be successful and achieve things. So we spend our lives striving to achieve more and more. We look for success, influence, money, and position, hoping that when we achieve those things, we will feel happy and accepted and loved by others.

We do not see how many people we ignore and reject in our desire to achieve our goals, which are not just those of business and career, but other goals of society, such as good relationships, happy marriages, children to be proud of, and a nice home. So we ignore the many whose opinion we consider unimportant, on the outside chance of being accepted by the few whose approval we value.

It is a poor exchange. Not only that, it doesn't work. Even when we achieve goals we have set our hearts on, we don't experience the satisfaction and fulfillment we imagined we would — or not for long. At first we may feel accepted, even loved, by those around us. Then we begin to see that often other people are making us feel good because they want something from us. The acceptance they show is not for us as people; it is for what we have achieved and what we possess. Many successful people find, at the end of their lives, that success is an illusion: it has not brought them happiness.

## Substituting Self-Acceptance
## for Approval

Even if we do experience true acceptance from others, it is still no substitute for self-acceptance and we will

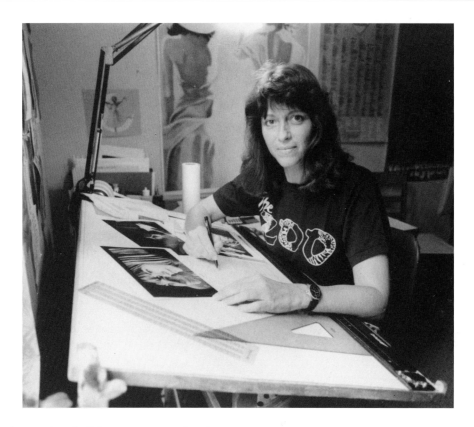

still feel unsatisfied and unfulfilled at a deeper level. We may feel that we are just not as successful as someone else or not as successful as we want to be. Until we learn to accept ourselves fully just as we are, no amount of external acceptance, approval, or love will make us truly happy.

One way to learn self-acceptance is through selfless service, Karma Yoga. Paradoxically, when we forget our own needs and serve others, we have a greater ability to accept ourselves and feel fulfilled and content with who we are and what we are doing with our lives.

Selfless service removes more than anxiety about the results of our actions. It also removes anxiety about whether we will receive enough for our services. We know from the start that material reward is not the main purpose; the main purpose is to help others. So satisfaction is received in every moment, as we are performing each action.

When we give more of ourselves to others through our work, we experience a deep sense of satisfaction and fulfillment. Not only do we feel more acceptance from others, but we also begin to accept ourselves because we know we are responding to our inborn desire to give to others. That is why wise men have always said that it is in giving that we receive: we receive the benefits of following our own pure, inner nature.

In selfless service we escape from the circle of the constant need to achieve and get credit for our actions in order to feel accepted. We no longer have to depend on someone else to accept and approve of us before we can accept and approve of ourselves.

It may not happen immediately just because we read and understand an article like this. For a while we may still find ourselves looking to others for approval. But gradually, as we practice making our work a service, we will move out of that stage into an even greater feeling of freedom and joy.

## Selfless Service: The Key to Lasting Happiness

Sometimes it may be hard to see our work as service to others; we may feel we don't have that kind of job. But all actions are service if they are inspiring to others. If we perform all our actions with total commitment, we are truly serving others because they will feel our energy and be inspired by it. When we do something with enthusiasm, sincerity, and detachment from the results, we ignite a flame of inspiration among those around us, and they love us for it.

The attitude of energetic commitment is what distinguishes the acceptance of Karma Yoga from mere passivity. Karma Yoga says that we are to do everything that we can, with total dedication and creativity, yet without feeling any anxiety about the results. That enthusiastic and energetic detachment is the key to true success in life — the success of lasting inner happiness, independent of all external events. That is the secret of Karma Yoga.

# TRANSFORMING WORK INTO SERVICE
## by Yogi Amrit Desai

In life we constantly strive for understanding, acceptance, and love from others. Yet often we find ourselves frustrated in our efforts. The more we fail to get what we need, the harder we try, until we create such a strong need to receive that we forget to give. The constant desire to receive is the greatest obstacle to receiving what we need. When we are selfish, we suffer the consequences of violating nature's most basic law of giving and receiving.

## Giving: The First Law of Nature

In the world of nature there is continuous exchange, a never-ending pattern of giving and receiving in which everything changes constantly and nothing remains stagnant. The ocean receives water from the sky only to give off water, which is then drawn up into the sky again. That water, transformed into rain, is given to rivers and eventually returns to the ocean.

The trees give their seeds to the earth, which nourishes and sustains them and eventually gives forth new trees. The continuous pattern of giving and receiving has only one exception: human beings, who alone violate that law and replace it with the unnatural laws of the individual ego.

When we violate nature's laws by receiving more than we give, the lost harmony of nature within us sends signals that an imbalance has been created. These signals come to us as feelings of fear, loneliness, frustration, or depression. Through each of those experiences, nature is trying to direct our attention to the basic disharmony we have created in and around us, through our unconscious selfishness.

## Taking: The First Law of Ego

Selfishness is the first law of the ego and the source of much of the conflict, separateness, and loneliness we experience. When selfishness arises, the light of love dissolves into the darkness of ignorance. No other form of ignorance can hurt as deeply. Selfishness says: "I want you to understand me, whether I understand you or not. I want you to accept me, whether I accept you or not. I want you to love me, whether I love you or not." It knows only one way: the way of receiving. It makes us blind to the needs of others. We see only ourselves; others are simply the means to fulfill our personal dreams.

This selfishness may even drive us to ignore, use, and ultimately hurt others in our attempt to fulfill our cherished dreams. Yet those dreams and desires can never be fully satisfied because we will never get enough. Once we are gripped in the jaws of our selfish desires, we ceaselessly strive for more while continuously working, out of fear, to protect what we already have.

In such striving there is no arriving — no point of satisfaction and satiation. Our consciousness has become caught in the vicious circle of endless wanting and endless striving.

## Trapped in the Web of Self-Interest

We do not do this intentionally, for we do not want to ignore or hurt others. Yet as soon as we experience a powerful desire for something, be it an external possession or position or a specific response from another, we automatically view others according to their ability to provide what we want.

Ironically, we are often the last to realize what we are doing. We play games without knowing that we play games. Others may recognize our games, but we ourselves are often unable to see them. So we become more deeply trapped in our own web of dishonesty and self-interest.

We find ourselves in greater and greater conflict with others, yet we are unable to recognize the source of the conflict as being within us. Such is the blindness of selfishness. Selfishness and loneliness are synonymous. When we are selfish, we feel alone and separate from others.

In order to feel the closeness that we need, we seek others' understanding of us; we try to win the understanding or acceptance of the other rather than to give to the other. Yet we also unconsciously realize that we will only get what we want from the other by appearing to be selfless in every possible way. We know that the other will accept and trust us to the degree that we appear to be selfless, so we put on the garb of selflessness.

## Our Secret List of Wants

When people first meet, they are usually wearing the garb of selflessness. Each gives to the other, thinking of what the other wants and striving to meet the needs of the other. But each person has two secret lists: a list of their own needs and a list of what they believe to be the other's needs.

If people think they will get what they want from the other, they act as though they can give the other what he or she wants. They don't put their own list first, but secretly they watch how the needs on their own list are being met.

Neither person is seeing the true characteristics of the other. Each sees only the facade that the other has adopted in order to make sure that his or her needs are met. The facade has been designed unconsciously and the real person hidden unintentionally, but eventually it becomes a habitual way of behaving.

When people are new to each other, they generally allow their own selfish needs to recede into the background. But habits are habits and cannot be hidden for long without a lot of strain and effort. So eventually people begin to let their own selfish needs come to the front again and conflict develops.

The dynamic happens as much in work relationships as in personal relationships. Most people are constantly trying to experience the joy of closeness with others and, at the same time, trying to keep their distance so that they can protect their own selfish dreams.

They fear that if they let others come too close, they will not be accepted as they really are. So we cannot live with each other, and yet we cannot live without each other either. We cannot tolerate closeness, yet we cannot bear the pain of feeling separate from others. So we live in constant inner conflict.

## The Solution: Selfless Service

The solution is to reduce our selfish desires and learn true selflessness, rather than putting on the appearance of selflessness. If you learn to give, receiving is already hidden in it. Such giving is an art. Only when you learn to give without expectation of return does your giving become instant receiving.

Receiving then begins even before you give because that kind of receiving happens inside you. You experience internally the rehearsal of your giving and you imagine how it will help, and your inner joy brings such a transformation in you that you begin to receive automatically and spontaneously even before you have given anything.

Such a deep joy in giving is the purest gift, one that very few are able to experience. So the true art of receiving what you really want is the art of giving. The following are six ways in which you can learn to be more selfless:

## Six Steps to Selfless Service

### 1. Recognize Others' Needs

Learning to be selfless is a lifelong practice. In the beginning you do not need to let go of all your wants; you simply need to recognize the needs of the other also. The first stage of learning selflessness is the willingness to have a fair exchange. At this stage you have a combination of selfishness and selflessness. You are selfish to a degree — you want something for yourself — but you also wish to give. And you begin to see others in terms of what they need, with compassion.

### 2. First, Accept Others' Selfishness

Your own selfishness will not be understood or accepted by others unless you are willing to understand and accept their selfishness. If both say "I want to be understood first," there is no meeting ground for either. Only by first being willing to accept the other's selfishness can you initiate the process by which the other can also accept it and become free of it, not by satisfying it but by understanding it.

Love and selfishness are diametrical opposites yet most people make constant efforts to mix both in every relationship. You want to get something out of the relationship and you also want it to be a loving relationship. It never happens, because selfishness is the invisible wall that separates you from love. The dawn of love is the death of selfishness.

### 3. Constantly Give Out the Love You Receive

You cannot receive unless you give. If you receive love and acceptance, you must constantly give it out in return. In the process of giving and receiving you are continuously being emotionally flushed out and all your impurities are washed away. If you only receive, you become clogged and unable to receive further.

If you fill your pail with water and neglect to empty it, the water will become stagnant and the pail will be unable to take in new, fresh water. In the same way, the container of love that is your heart cannot cling to the love it receives without becoming stagnant. You must be ready to give out the love you receive.

### 4. Give More than You Think You Are Receiving

Selfishness is the source of many conflicts and misunderstandings. The whole purpose of personal or spiritual growth is to learn to let go of selfishness and gradually become able to give. As you progress in this learning process you must go past the stage of fair exchange and gradually become willing to have an unfair exchange. Willingness must exist for any relationship to work, because as long as

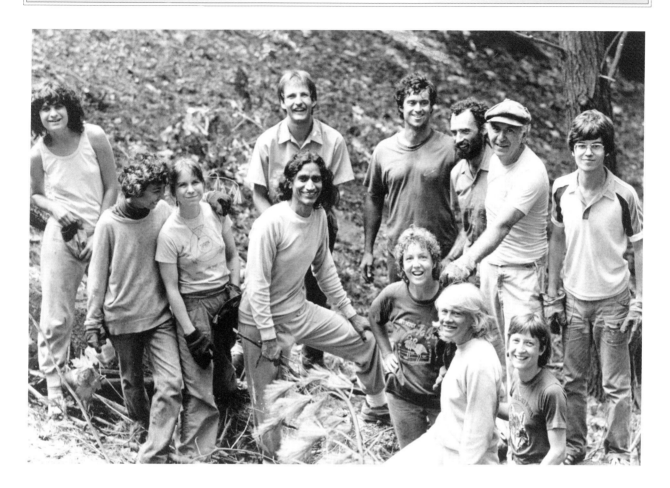

both people expect a fair exchange, each one remains focused on the unfairness of the other. One person must be willing to have a bad deal if love is to last. You must be willing to be cheated, consciously knowing what you are doing, realizing what is happening as you let go. Then your losing becomes winning, because now your entire value system is different.

### 5. Serve without Seeking Any Return

The benefit of service is not in getting what you want, but in consciously learning to let go of your selfishness. As you experience letting go, you begin to see that receiving happens for you in a very strange way. Externally you may not receive anything, yet internally you begin to receive the essence of all you really want, which is peace, comfort, and fulfillment. Externally you may have even lost a great deal, but internally you receive the results of success as you experience satisfaction, contentment, and joy.

Service is a very direct and simple way to learn selflessness. The basic idea behind service is that you give without asking for a return. Such service is the antidote to conflict, the antidote to separateness, loneliness, and fear of the other.

Service is an unfailing tool that invariably shows you where you are being egotistical and not truly giving. Most conflicts you come across as you serve are the direct outcome of your own selfishness. If in the past you have been excessively selfish, you will encounter more conflicts in service.

They are not new conflicts. You are simply beginning to see the conflicts and selfishness that has been buried inside you, and service is the mirror that allows you to see. The purpose of seeing your selfishness is to enable you gradually to become free through understanding.

### 6. Serve in Areas in Which You Seek Growth

In deciding where you will offer your service there is one basic principle to follow: choose the source from which you wish to receive. Once you begin to give your service, you will invariably begin to receive from that source also, because it is impossible to separate giving and receiving.

If you give service or even financial support to an organization you become subtly connected to that organization and the effects of its work return to you in a variety of ways. You become part of whomever you serve.

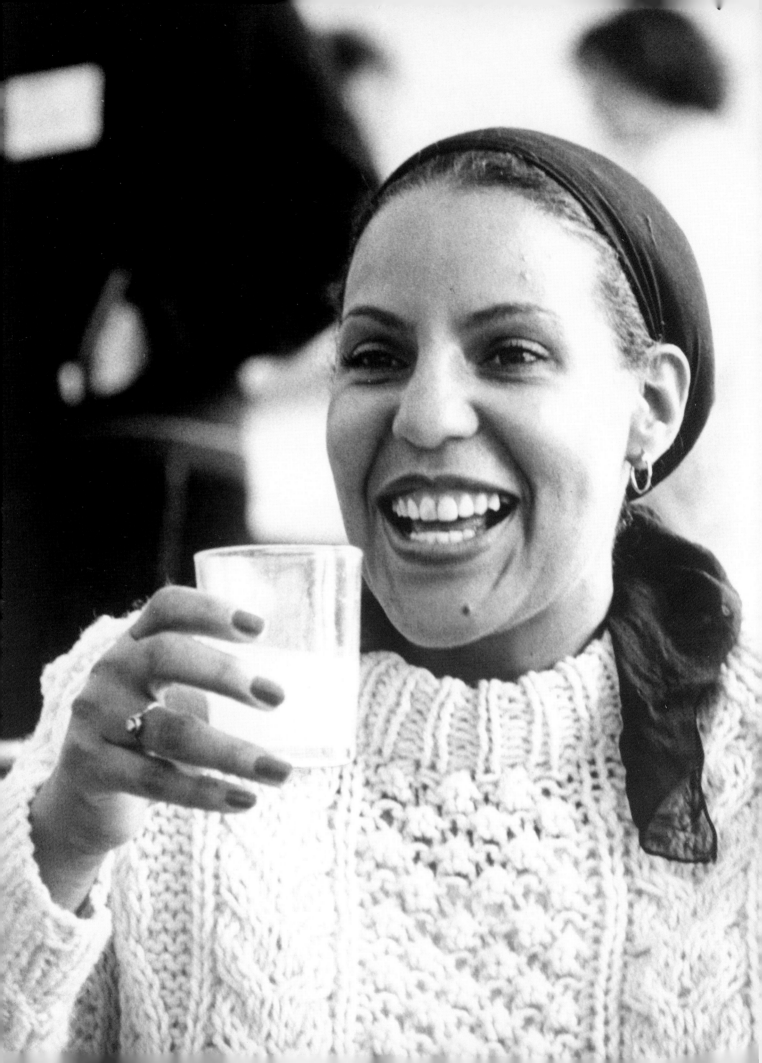

# The Fifth Pathway

## discovering your optimum diet

# Eating Well — Your Way

There are so many books and magazines about diet and nutrition on the market that one of them is aptly titled *Are You Confused?* Certainly, many people are confused. Most of those books and articles have been written by sincerely motivated people, many of whom are experts whose theories are based on scientific findings and sound experimentation, yet they seem to disagree on all but the most fundamental facts.

So whom are we to believe? Why is there so much disagreement? How are we to know what really is the best, most nutritious diet for us? How can we learn to discriminate between the many options available and find our own optimum diet? This chapter addresses those questions.

The Kripalu Approach does not recommend one diet over another, for most have merit. Instead, it teaches an approach to nutrition that enables you to become free forever of diets and nutrition plans devised by other people. It will give you the liberating experience of becoming your own nutritional expert by learning to hear the messages of your personal, inner diet doctor, your prana.

The emphasis is on you and your personal experience. With that in mind, start off by completing the Self-Discovery Experience that follows. It may lead you to a totally new perspective on eating.

After that, you will find we have separated the discussion on nutrition into two distinct areas. The first is the conventional one, focusing on what you eat and reviewing the kinds of foods that are beneficial (and not so beneficial) to health. The second area of discussion is special to the Kripalu Approach. It focuses on how and why you eat, which is a key area that is missing from so many other approaches to diet and nutrition.

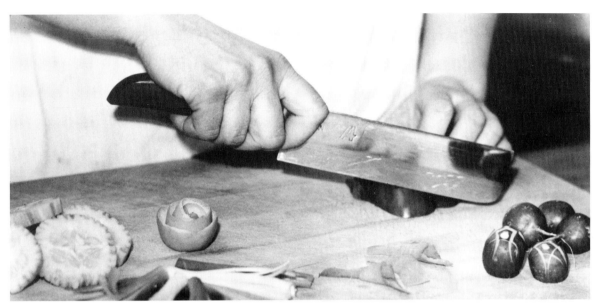

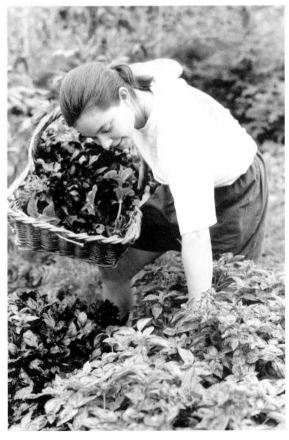

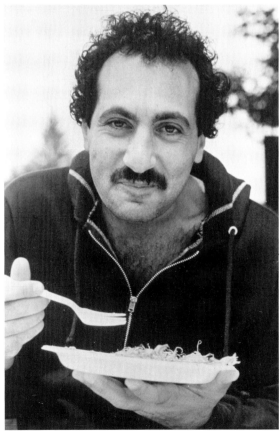

## Self-Discovery Experience

## 12

### What can you learn from your eating patterns?

### Awareness

1. Sit quietly with your eyes closed. Then, without directing or judging them, begin to let thoughts and associations connected with food and eating flow through your mind. Simply let the thoughts happen and write them down in brief catch phrases or draw them. Close your eyes again and allow more to come. Do that for about five minutes.

2. See yourself going through a typical day and visualize all the times that you stopped to take any form of food or drink, whether it was a meal or a snack. Consciously recall for each instance how you were feeling, what you were thinking and doing before, during, and after the meal, snack, or drink. Notice particularly whether you were calm and relaxed, tense, tired, emotional, hungry, bored, or whatever. Write down or draw each of those "food events" as you recall them. (For example: "At 11 A.M., ate a doughnut and drank coffee — needed a break from work.")

## Acceptance

3. Reread, item by item, what you have written thus far, objectively noting anything that you observe, recognize, or learn from what you see. Just write down what comes to mind, without puzzling over it too much or criticizing it.

4. Using the questions below to begin the process, look for habit patterns that may currently govern your eating. Be honest, but accepting; do not judge what you see as good or bad — simply acknowledge the patterns for what they are.

   (a) How often do I eat from real, physical hunger and how often from habit, a desire for pleasurable taste sensations, or other desires, such as combating boredom, consoling myself, or taking away or dissipating negative emotions such as fear, anger, or depression?

   (b) How often do I eat slowly, peacefully, and quietly in relaxed surroundings? How often do I eat on the run, hurriedly, with tension or anger, while discussing or arguing, while reading, listening to the radio, or watching TV, or involved in some other activity?

   (c) How often do I really taste and enjoy what I eat, and how often do I find I've eaten a whole meal almost without noticing?

   (d) How often do I stop when I know I've had enough, and how often do I go on eating because it tastes so good, because I don't want to go back to what I need to do after eating, or because I have nothing else to do?

   (e) How often do I feel alert and pleasantly satisfied after a meal and how often do I feel uncomfortably full, have indigestion, or feel sleepy and dull?

   (f) How often do I eat healthy, nutritious, live foods and how often do I "junk out" on artificial, processed, sweet, carbohydrate-heavy, or nutritionless foods?

Go over all that you have written so far and try to observe some typical patterns in your eating. Are there specific times of day, days of the week, or situations where you can observe yourself eating less well than at other times? Note those patterns and write them down.

## Adjustment

Read the section called "How to Cultivate the Art of Conscious Eating" and choose some ways in which you can begin to change your eating habits so that they are more conducive to health and well-being. Start in small ways — perhaps relaxing for a few minutes before each meal, cutting back on the amount of coffee you drink, or deciding to snack less between meals. Just begin to be aware.

Watch what you eat and how and when you eat, and see what more you can learn from that information. Most of all, drop any feelings of guilt you have about eating "wrongly." It's better to eat the "wrong" thing with relaxation and enjoyment than to feel guilty and self-rejecting about it. Perhaps it is even better than eating the right thing with resentment, longing, or tension. No matter what, feel good about yourself.

# Finding Which Foods
# Are Just Right for You

## You Are Unique

Among the many diet and nutrition books on the market, there is none superior to our own body when it comes to finding our personal, optimum diet for physical, mental, and spiritual well-being. The reasons that the wide range of books and diet programs available often ends up creating confusion, rather than clarity, are several.

First, the authors wrote at different times and places for different people and cultures. Second, no matter how well-schooled the author, he or she is still interpreting the facts through a set of personal, subjective, experiential filters. Third, everyone is different: a book or diet has, of necessity, been developed based on the "average" person, and the average person simply does not exist. Each person's nutritional requirement is different because his or her history, metabolism, and energy needs are unique.

## Prana:
## Your Own Inner Nutrition Specialist

The ultimate answer is to learn to rely on our inner body wisdom or prana for guidance. As we have seen, most of us have forgotten how to read the signals of prana. We don't even hear it until it shouts at us through the unmistakable language of pain, and then frequently our first response is trying to eliminate the pain by taking remedies — antacids, painkillers, and such — rather than seeing the pain as a messenger and learning to understand what it is saying.

That is where the Kripalu Approach differs from others. Rather than prescribing another set of food rules, it teaches us two things: (1) how to tune in to that personal, inner nutrition specialist called prana, and (2) how to interpret what prana teaches.

How can you relearn this lost ability to communicate with your prana about the food your body needs? It can be accomplished by informed and guided personal experimentation. There are two distinct stages in this process of arriving at a personal diet that is optimally supportive of holistic health.

The first stage is transitional. While learning to develop an informed sensitivity to your body's needs, it is still necessary to follow a set of externally proposed guidelines for appropriate nutrition, but always with flexibility and as great an awareness as possible.

At this stage, the signals you perceive will often be misleading. They may be caused by habitual desires and preferences rather than by genuine bodily needs. You may crave something sweet, for instance, when your body really needs protein.

You graduate to the second stage when you have learned to interpret the language of your body well. Then you can listen confidently to your own prana and develop the diet that is uniquely suited to you and no one else.

## Your Food Is Your Medicine

Many ancient peoples knew that food is medicine — not just because herbs can be used to cure various ills, but because the proper diet helps to keep the body in a constant state of optimal health. Ancient India's Ayurvedic system of medicine was based on that belief, and yoga has always taught that our level of consciousness is determined in part by what we put into our bodies.

Modern science has discovered that every single cell in the human body is replaced over a period of seven years and that these new cells are made up of the nourishment we have taken into our bodies. So we are, literally, what we eat.

To understand how your food affects your consciousness, you need to learn what happens to the food that you take into your body. There are three scenarios: Some food is digested and then turned into either fuel for the body or new tissue. Some is excreted. Some is retained in the body, yet is useless. The useless food may become fatty deposits, which are usually highly visible, but it may also linger as toxic material lodged invisibly in or around the cells of the body, sapping vitality, fogging the mind and emotions, and causing disease and premature aging.

## Prana and Purification

There are two ways to eliminate those toxins from the body: (1) purifying your diet so that you take in only what you need and can use or excrete, and (2) purifying your body of accumulated toxins and waste products.

Purifying the diet must be done gradually, so as not to shock your system too much, for the body is a creature of habit and likes its familiar foods. It is necessary for this purification process to know two things: (a) which foods are generally agreed, by most sources, to be harmful, and (b) the general effect on the body-mind of different types of food.

In the category of harmful foods come additives of all kinds, refined products such as white flour and white sugar, and red meats. Some say all animal flesh is harmful; however, a transition diet can include moderate amounts of poultry and fish. Meat is better avoided because it often contains harmful substances, such as hormones fed to fatten the animals and adrenaline released by their fear at the moment of death. Both are unhealthy for humans.

There are many stages to dietary purification; many vegetarians come to a stage where they wish to eliminate all dairy products, but that is an optional later stage.

## Diet and Energy

It is useful to know that certain kinds of food provide specific types of energy to your body. A little self-observation will illustrate that.

Rich, heavy foods (such as many pasta dishes, steaks with rich sauces, breads, and pastries and cakes) will tend to leave you feeling rather heavy and lethargic, as will alcohol, when the first rush of energy has faded.

Highly spiced foods, coffee, and black tea are examples of foods that will leave you feeling energetic, yet often restless and irritable.

Most fruits, vegetables, and whole grains will leave you feeling balanced, calm, clear-headed, and relaxed.

If you simply observe how you feel after eating, you will be able to choose your foods accordingly. The signals to look for after a meal are "fogginess" and difficulty in concentrating, tiredness, irritability, unexplained emotions, and over-reactions. Watch for patterns and try to relate them to your eating. Some signals may not appear until the day after you ate whatever caused them.

The complex combinations of food we eat may confuse the issue. We tend to eat lethargy-inducing food along with restless-energy food and often have the illusion of a balanced result. A typical heavy, rich meal followed by coffee is a good example.

What is actually happening when we combine foods that way is that we are depleting the body's store of energy as it struggles to balance two conflicting inputs. For specific guidance on which foods to avoid combining, see the Food Combination Chart in this section.

Another rule, then, for healthy eating is to keep it simple, especially while trying to observe which foods are pleasing and acceptable to your body and which are less so.

Part of what leads us into miscombinations is our tendency to eat to please our tongues, rather than our whole body-mind. We eat what tempts our palate, in quantities that please our appetite. Those preferences are usually stimulated by habit or emotion, rather than by our bodies' true nutritional needs and our digestive and eliminative capacity. The latter messages are more subtle.

To eat for health, we need to listen more to the actual needs of our bodies. Of course, none of us can expect to break habits overnight; our awareness and understanding is sure to come faster than our ability or even our desire to change. That's normal. But we can at least begin to balance the choices that result from desires and cravings with those that are consciously more healthful. That will be a fine start.

## Food Selection Guidelines

### Foods to Select

Fresh fruit and dried fruit

Fresh vegetables

Fruit or vegetable juices

Sprouted seeds and legumes (alfalfa, lentil, chickpea, sesame, sunflower, peanut)

Nuts and seeds

Beans and legumes

Whole grains and cereals

Whole grain bread

Honey, blackstrap molasses, maple syrup, rice syrup, barley malt

Herbal teas and coffee substitutes

Tofu and other soy products

Milk and dairy products, in moderation

### Foods to Avoid

Canned or processed foods

Refined sugar or sugar products

Artificial preservatives or additives

Refined flour products

Overcooked foods

Meat

Animal oils and fats

#### Non-foods to Avoid

Caffeine

Alcohol

Drugs, unless vital

# Fasting

The second stage of purification is the elimination of already existing physical impurities. Vigorous physical exercise has long been recognized as a good way to burn off not only excess calories, but also toxic wastes. Jogging, cycling, regular swimming, racquet sports, yoga, and other activities are all excellent ways to exercise the body and rid it of toxic food deposits.

Another powerful way to speed up the elimination of toxins is periodic fasting. In ages past, almost every culture has advocated fasting because of its effectiveness.

The term fasting can describe many different levels of non-regular eating, not just living on water. There are two major benefits of fasting: It gives the digestive system time to rest and repair itself, rather than working around the clock as it usually does, and it enables the body to eliminate toxic wastes.

Only when the body ceases the digestive process does detoxification occur. Normally, great amounts of body energy (some estimates say up to sixty-five percent after a heavy meal) are consumed in digesting our food. A moderately heavy meal requires about six hours of work from organs such as the heart, kidneys, and liver, and even more from the digestive organs. It takes anywhere from twenty-four to seventy hours for one meal to pass through the body.

When we fast, the energy usually claimed by digestion is freed for a thorough housecleaning of the system. The body becomes lighter and more flexible; the mind becomes clear and more creative. Greater intuitive powers may develop and deep spiritual insights may be experienced after a period of time. A feeling of well-being arises when the energy is freed in this way: problems suddenly become solutions and ideas begin to flow.

The Kripalu Approach advocates a form of fasting adapted from traditional yogic fasting. It involves taking only fruit, fruit juice, or freshly pressed vegetable juice for one or more days. We seldom recommend fasting on water alone, as this can cause unpleasant side effects in those not accustomed to fasting. Also, we have found that certain juices, particularly citrus and apple, are very cleansing and yet provide nourishment at the same time.

Fresh vegetable juices are even easier for the novice faster: the cleansing is less intense and more nourishment is provided for rebuilding and replacing cells. We generally recommend taking fresh citrus fruit or juice for breakfast, and vegetable juice at lunch and for supper.

Fasting in this way, on a regular basis, definitely leads to greater physical health. One day per week (preferably the same day) is ideal, but if you can't manage that try fasting once every two to four weeks. From time to time a longer fast (three to four days) is beneficial , particularly at the change of seasons. It helps the body's adaptive processes.

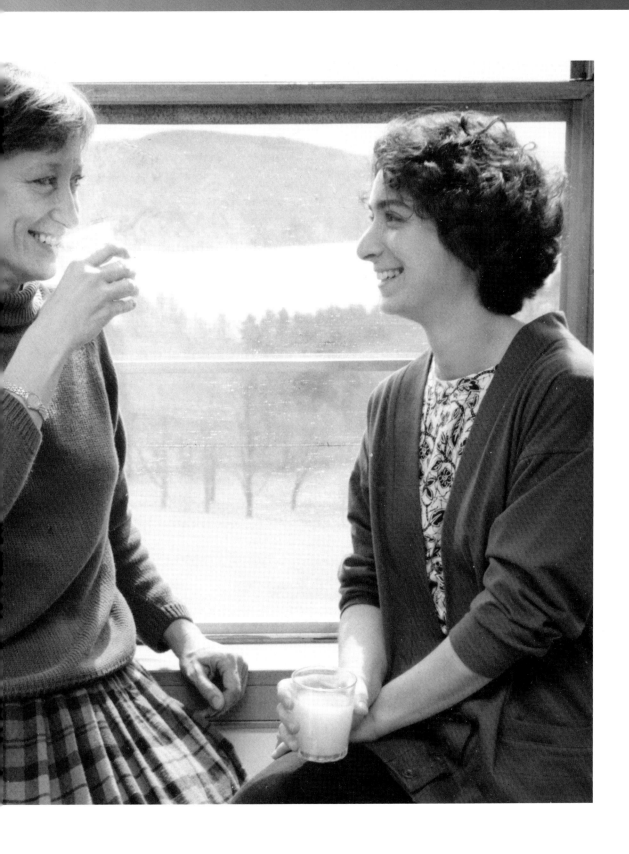

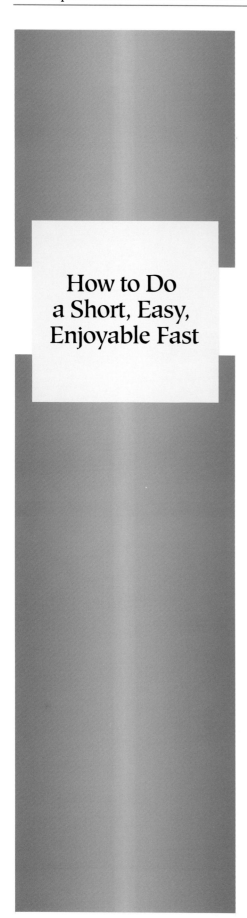

# How to Do a Short, Easy, Enjoyable Fast

## Preparation

Short fasts are extremely beneficial and not difficult for persons of average health. Some factors should be considered, however, such as age, physical condition, weight, and the nature of any work that must go on during the fast.

An appropriate medical expert should be consulted before a fast or purification diet is undertaken by young children, or those who are underweight or have low blood pressure or blood sugar. Even healthy people should consult a fasting specialist before attempting a fast of over five days, so that they know how to deal with metabolic changes that may result.

If you are a meat-eater or if your system is highly toxic, you will find it helpful to prepare for your fast by gradually reducing your intake of meat and substituting a greater variety of wholesome vegetarian foods for a few months. Do this in stages. First, reduce your intake of meat. Then, select one day each week on which you will eat only salad. That will hasten the purification process. Continue with a one-day salad diet each week for at least eight weeks, and then begin eating fruit one day per week (only one kind of fruit on that day). After several weeks of fruit fasting you will be comfortable graduating to juice.

Eat a light dinner on the evening before a one-day fast. If you plan to fast for more than one day (which is not advised for a first fast), gradually reduce your intake of food over a period of several days before beginning the fast and eat only fruit and salads on the day immediately preceding.

## During Your Fast

Fast on only one kind of fruit or fruit juice (rather than combining fruits). Combinations of fruit, such as acid and sweet fruits, do not digest well together and create toxins within the system. Fruits such as apples, grapes, and citrus fruits are very cleansing. Bananas are not recommended for fasting, as they are very starchy and not cleansing in nature.

When fasting on juice be sure to drink fresh vegetable juices or pure fruit juices to which no sugar has been added. Fruit juices that are recommended are apple, grape, orange, and grapefruit. If the juice is too concentrated for your taste, dilute it with water.

Drink plenty of water throughout the day, as water allows the circulation to flow more freely, accelerating the purification process occurring in the blood and kidneys.

Avoid coffee or caffeine-containing teas. Herbal teas or caffeine-free coffee are fine, but without any sweetener, even honey.

As your body begins to cleanse itself, you may experience some discomfort. The pores of your skin will eliminate many toxins, possibly causing body odor. As your lungs eliminate poisons, you may experience bad breath. Your tongue may become coated with a white coating, indicating that cleansing is taking place within your body.

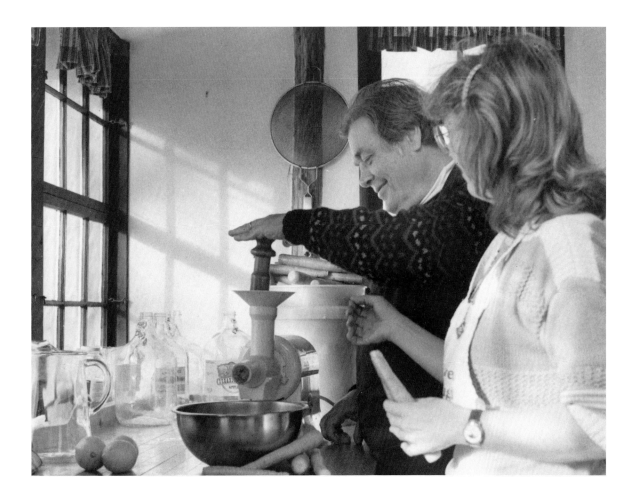

In the very early stages of fasting you may experience a slight headache, nausea, or cold chills. If those symptoms produce a lot of discomfort, eat a small amount of light food such as a salad, or switch to vegetable juice if you are on fruit juice, and remember that those discomforts are a good sign.

The more discomfort you feel, the better the fast is working: the more the body is cleansing itself. Such symptoms are caused by toxins being poured into your bloodstream as a result of the increased purification taking place in your body.

After some fasting experience, your body will become cleaner and you will be able to fast without any feeling of discomfort or tiredness. In fact, as your body purifies, you will gain energy during a fast, particularly after a few days of continuous fasting. You will begin to feel vigorous, energetic, creative, clear, and emotionally balanced.

As a result of fasting, many of the impurities thrown off by the organs are deposited in the intestines. Since your bowel movements will be reduced because you are not taking in any bulk, you need to take special measures to eliminate those impurities.

An effective way to cleanse the colon is to take an enema on the evening of a one-day fast and as needed during longer fasts. (See specific instructions later in this chapter.) Saunas are also beneficial to facilitate elimination of toxins.

Fast with an understanding and awareness of why you are fasting and keep your mind busy so that it does not dwell on food. If, while fasting, you continually think of food, you are not fasting but starving, and you will feel deprived and unhappy.

Cultivate a positive mental attitude by reading inspiring books and articles about the benefits of fasting. Direct your awareness to the changes taking place in your body and be happy and proud of what you are doing to purify and rejuvenate it and to attune more to prana.

# Experimenting with a Vegetarian Diet

More and more people from all walks of life are discovering the advantages of a vegetarian diet. Many newspapers and magazines report that athletes say they feel lighter and have more energy on a vegetarian diet, runners claim that they run faster and experience less muscle tension, movie stars find that it improves their skin and helps them stay more relaxed, writers and artists say they feel more clear-headed and creative, and many others simply find that they feel better and that it costs less.

## Your Ancestors Were Vegetarians

Science is finding increasing evidence that the earliest human beings ate a vegetarian diet and only turned to meat for survival when their vegetable sources disappeared. Carnivorous animals have relatively short digestive tracts, and the total time it takes for food to move through their body is relatively short. Animal flesh putrifies rather rapidly in the warm, moist environment of the body; the rapid digestion and elimination of carnivorous animals prevents that.

Animals that survive on plants have much longer intestinal tracts to allow for the breakdown of cellulose in the plant matter. Human beings have very long digestive systems — the intestines alone measure about thirty feet in length! When meat is processed through such a long tract, there is plenty of time for it to putrefy and spread toxins throughout the body.

As noted earlier, those of us in so-called civilized societies apparently now have such sluggish digestive and eliminative systems that it takes anywhere up to seventy-two hours for us to process and eliminate our food; in primitive societies the average length of time is twelve to thirty-six hours: a much healthier time span.

Teeth are another indicator of natural diet. Carnivorous animals have sharp, pointed teeth for tearing flesh; vegetarian animals have blunter teeth for grinding. We humans have only two sharp, pointed teeth, the so-called eye teeth. Many scientists feel that is another indication that we began our evolution as vegetarians.

Anthropologists examining the teeth of ancient humans by using a recently discovered and sophisticated method have reported that the pattern of wear on those teeth (as compared to that on animal teeth of the same period) was almost certainly caused by the eating of fruits and vegetables, not meat.

## Eating Vegetables Is Eating Sunshine

A vegetarian diet is highly suitable for human beings for many other reasons. Vegetables get their energy from the earth, from water, and from sunshine. They are high in vitamins and minerals and, as a primary form of food, can be eaten and digested easily. Meat, on the other hand, is inefficiently converted from plant life. Its molecules are complex and hard to digest. While meat is high in protein, it is low in many of the vitamins and minerals essential to man.

An increasing number of authorities now believe that many health problems are caused by the toxicity arising from the high uric acid and saturated fat content of meat. Excess uric acid is deposited and accumulated in various organs, causing diseases such as gout and rheumatism. Saturated fats are believed to cause blood pressure problems and hardening of the arteries.

Also, many animals are fed food that has been sprayed with pesticides that are retained in the fatty tissues of the animals and ingested along with the meat.

## Transition Diets

A vegetarian diet is not made up solely of vegetables. It includes a variety of foods, such as fresh fruits, nuts, beans, and grains. A "pure" vegetarian diet excludes all kinds of meat, fish, and poultry, as well as foods containing any form of animal life, such as eggs and dairy products.

There are modified vegetarian diets that do include such foods as fish, eggs, and dairy products. Those are good transition diets for people who have been meat-eaters all their lives. If you decide to experiment with reducing the amount of meat in your diet, be sure to do it gradually, as a sudden change might be a shock to your system.

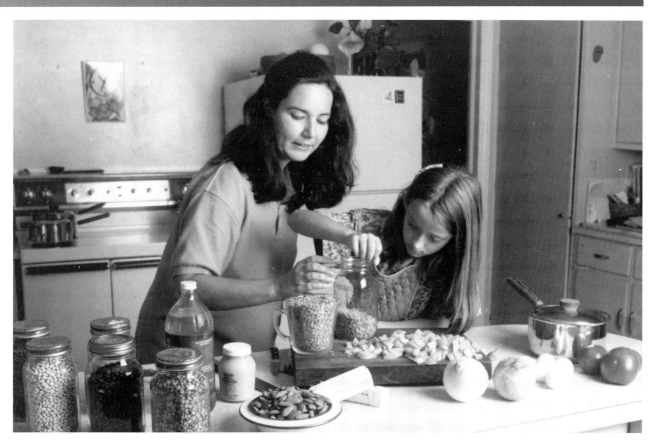

It is important when switching to a vegetarian menu to be certain you continue to get a balanced diet that contains ample protein. Recent research indicates that Americans do not need nearly so much protein as they are currently eating, however, or believe they need. Most eat sixty to seventy grams of protein a day, whereas recent studies, supported by historical evidence of societies with lower protein intake, show that thirty to forty grams is plenty.

Vegetarian protein sources are at least the equal of, and some say superior to, animal protein and are easy to include in the average person's diet. Dairy products, whole grains, and seeds and legumes (particularly sprouted ones) are good sources of protein. Soy products are excellent, especially tofu (sometimes called bean curd).

There are also some good natural supplements. We particularly recommend brewer's yeast for extra protein and for many of the B-vitamins sometimes lacking in a vegetarian diet, kelp for iodine and trace minerals, and unsulfured blackstrap molasses for iron and minerals.

That is a brief overview of vegetarian eating. Those seriously considering experimenting with a vegetarian diet would do well to read some of the excellent books available on the market and to consult with knowledgeable experts to avoid any stress in transition.

## STOP!

How aware are you of your body messages right now? How are you feeling? Is there tension, stiffness, or tiredness in any part of your body? Do you need to get up and stretch? Take some deep breaths? Relax your shoulders?  Rest your eyes? Rest your mind? Close your eyes for a minute and take some long, slow, deep breaths to enable you to get in touch with your experience. Then respond to what your body is asking you to do.

# FOOD COMBINING CHART

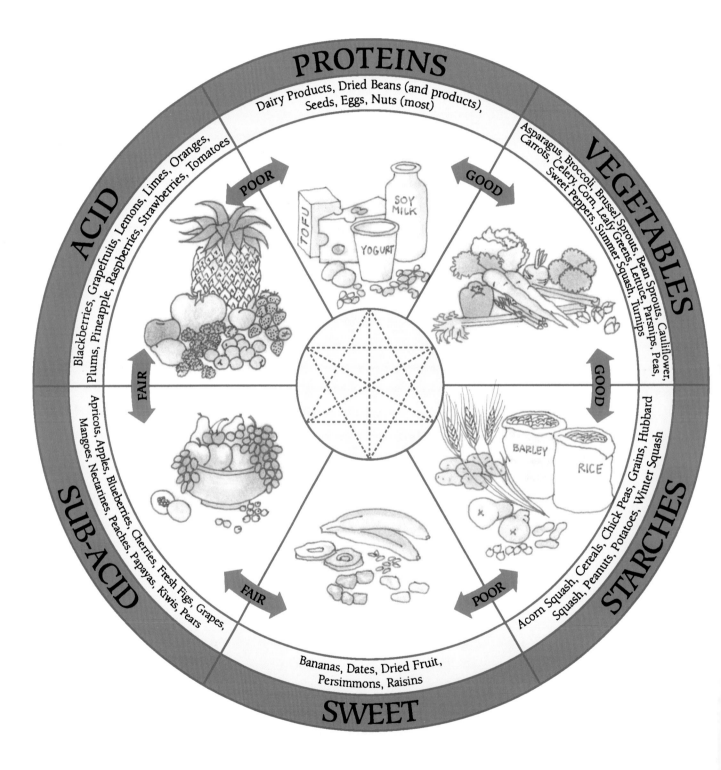

**PROTEINS**
Dairy Products, Dried Beans (and products), Seeds, Eggs, Nuts (most)

**VEGETABLES**
Asparagus, Broccoli, Brussel Sprouts, Cauliflower, Carrots, Celery, Corn, Leafy Greens, Lettuce, Parsnips, Peas, Sweet Peppers, Summer Squash, Turnips

**ACID**
Blackberries, Grapefruits, Lemons, Limes, Oranges, Plums, Pineapple, Raspberries, Strawberries, Tomatoes

**STARCHES**
Acorn Squash, Cereals, Chick Peas, Grains, Hubbard Squash, Peanuts, Potatoes, Winter Squash

**SUB-ACID**
Apricots, Apples, Blueberries, Cherries, Fresh Figs, Grapes, Mangoes, Nectarines, Peaches, Papayas, Kiwis, Pears

**SWEET**
Bananas, Dates, Dried Fruit, Persimmons, Raisins

POOR

GOOD

GOOD

FAIR

FAIR

POOR

All non-adjacent combinations
(indicated by dotted lines)
are poor combinations.

# EATING CONSCIOUSLY
## by Yogi Amrit Desai

## How Relaxation Affects Appetite

A major cause of inappropriate eating is hidden tension. Whenever you experience unpleasant emotions or feel tense, you are losing prana or energy. Then you unconsciously feel the need to replace that lost energy by eating.

Unfortunately, when you don't eat wisely, you lose more energy processing the food than you gain from the food, and a low-energy cycle is created. Such a cycle can be broken at several places.

First, if you learn to be more relaxed, you will need less food because there is less lost energy to be replenished. When you are very tense, you may eat three or four large meals a day and still feel hungry. If you are relaxed, one or two light meals may be sufficient.

Second, you can improve your eating patterns so that digestion does not drain the energy you gained from the food. And third, you can understand and change the tension-related attitudes that affect your eating habits.

When we are tense, we tend to seek relaxation and fulfillment through gratifying our senses. Food is the fastest and easiest way to do that. Actually, our search for pleasure and enjoyment through food, entertainment, fun, and sexual relationships, is often hiding an inner emptiness that comes from spiritual starvation — from not feeling fulfilled on all levels of our being. Usually we recognize only our physical lack of fulfillment, however.

Western society is very food oriented, with resulting problems of overeating and poor digestion. Television advertising reflects that very accurately: Commercials for delicious-looking foods are almost immediately followed by commercials for antacids and digestive aids, or for the latest fads in reducing diets!

## Rediscovering Natural Hunger

Because of this excessive food orientation and the constant seeking of taste sensations to satisfy ourselves superficially and dull our inner yearnings, we have overstimulated our appetites to the point where we can no longer hear the real inner physical needs of our bodies.

Instead, the appetite we hear and respond to is the one produced by our minds and our desires for taste sensations. Those desires are simply our wish to repeat previous experiences; they are habits based on memories of previously pleasurable tastes. So we have developed eating habits that detract from, rather than contribute to, our health and well-being.

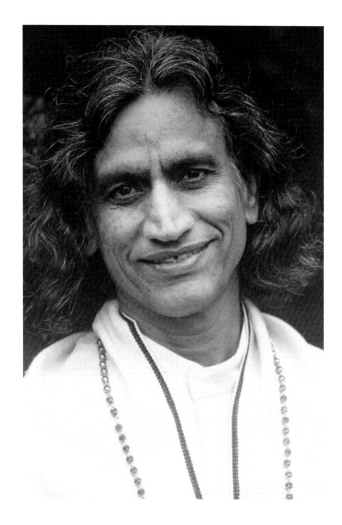

Often we eat when we are not really hungry, in the sense of having a naturally stimulated physical hunger. You know from experience that when you have been very active physically out in fresh air, you have such a healthy appetite that even the simplest foods taste wonderfully satisfying. When you have been sitting at a desk all day in a busy office, even the most delicious meal may not fully satisfy.

When we cannot experience the complete satisfaction that comes from eating with natural hunger, we often seek artificial ways to gain that satisfaction. We eat foods that are elaborately prepared, exotic, and rich, with unusual tastes, exciting colors, and textures. We try to stimulate hunger artificially, with little "appetizers" and a variety of alcoholic "aperitifs." Of course, neither the additives that are needed to create such foods nor the alcohol contribute to health. Satisfaction comes from how much genuine hunger we experience, not from the elaborate taste or texture of what we consume.

The loss of natural hunger is also the cause of most overeating. We have seen that when we are tense and not able to enjoy our lives fully, we seek pleasure from eating. But because of our unhealthy, physically inactive lifestyles, we cannot derive full satisfaction from the food we eat, so we seek a greater level of satisfaction by eating more and more, which creates another unhealthy cycle.

## Are You Eating to Live — or Living to Eat?

At the root of the problem lies the fact that many people have forgotten the true role of eating in life. Eating is first of all to provide nourishment and sustain our life processes so that we can explore and develop our higher potentials. We have distorted that basic function of food and made it primarily a means to satisfy our senses of taste and smell.

If we forget that primary purpose of eating, but consume food that is basically healthy, we will still be likely to damage our health by overeating or combining our foods unwisely. What is available in natural food stores today is ready proof of that. Those stores are full of a broad selection of "natural," "healthy," "organic" delicacies and treats, all packaged to tempt the palate!

So you still run the danger of over-indulging or eating poorly, even with health foods, unless you remain conscious of your true purpose in eating. You must eat to nourish your body, because it is, as many sages have said, the temple of the soul.

Remember that "natural" does not necessarily mean best. Even natural foods need to be eaten with discrimination. Create your diet in accordance with what you know from experience is best for your health. Eat in accordance with your prana. Most of all, become conscious of your motivations for eating. As you cultivate attitudes toward eating that are more supportive of your health, you will receive immediate benefits: you will enjoy your food more and gain a richer experience of health and well-being in your life.

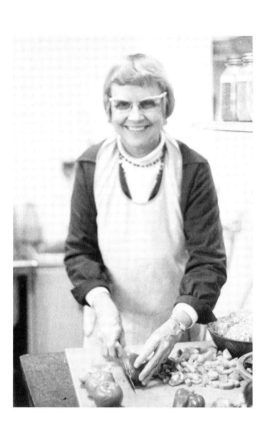

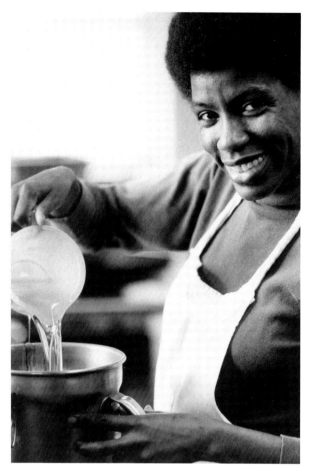

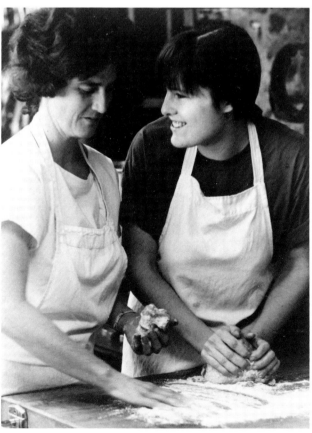

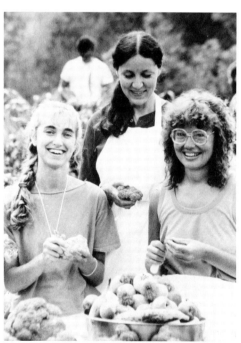

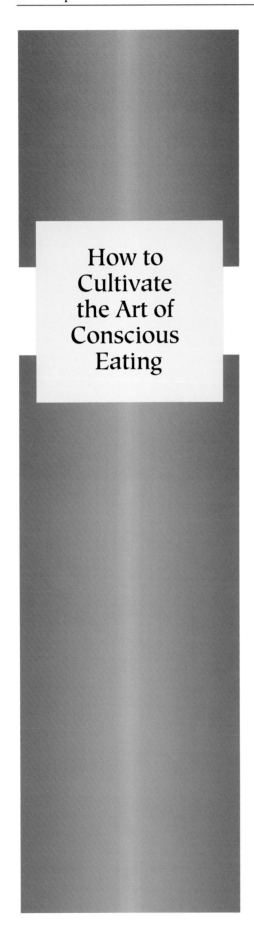

# How to Cultivate the Art of Conscious Eating

What does conscious eating mean? It means eating with full awareness of where, how, and why, as well as what, you are eating. It means slowing down and paying attention — really being present. It means devoting your full attention, during a meal, to the actual process of eating, so as to obtain both maximum health benefits and maximum enjoyment. Here's how to cultivate the art:

1. Eat only when you are hungry. Even if you eat more than someone else, it will benefit you as long as you are hungry. If you do not seem to be getting much joy out of eating at a particular moment or are dissatisfied with the variety of food available, either you are not really hungry or you are eating more than your natural appetite requires. When you are hungry, the simplest food tastes the most delicious.

   After eating, you should feel relaxed and alert. If you feel tired or sluggish, you know that you have eaten too much. When you eat less, you may experience hunger at first. That is because any change from habit will give rise to an initial protest from the body, but that protest comes from the previous times when you have overeaten or eaten improperly, not from having missed a meal or two.

   The initial discomfort that comes from getting to know true hunger is caused by the body beginning to purify, which is a positive, healthy process. Hunger is a gift of nature. It is an expression of prana, our inner physician. When you allow yourself to become truly hungry, then eating is an exquisite pleasure, a natural fulfillment of a real bodily need.

2. Eat regularly at specific times. Plan each meal and eat a quantity such that you will again be hungry by the time of your next meal. In that way, you will eat only when you are hungry and you will eat regularly as well.

3. Focus all your attention on what is happening in your mouth as you chew. That has two benefits: First, you will chew thoroughly. That is important because a significant portion of the digestive process is accomplished by enzymes secreted in the mouth. If you do not chew properly, you are bypassing that important stage of digestion and forcing your stomach to compensate by working harder than nature intended. Chronic indigestion, gas, and constipation will result.

   Second, if you really pay attention to your chewing, you will gain such taste satisfaction from your food that you will not need to overeat.

4. Select the proper amount and type of food for your individual system. This will vary according to your age, weight, sex, and the type of work you do. Strenuous physical work requires a heavier diet; sedentary work is done more efficiently when eating lightly.

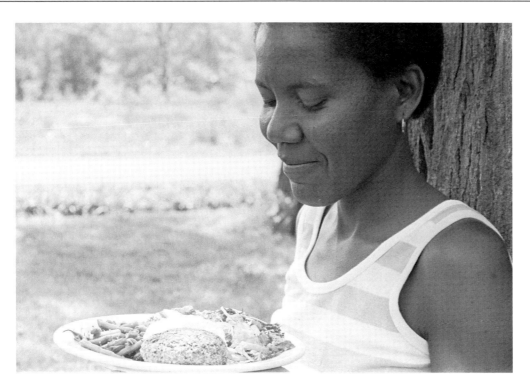

5.  Avoid eating when you are angry, excited, tense, depressed, sick, hurried, or tired. Wait until your mind becomes calm and your natural hunger returns. The hunger you experience when tense is not true hunger. It is mentally induced hunger, designed to provide an outlet for your nervousness and anxieties. True hunger arises only when you are relaxed.

6.  Always eat in a pleasant atmosphere. Make your meals attractive and your place of eating pleasant and soothing. Begin your meal with a simple prayer or by observing a moment of silence to reflect with gratitude upon the gift of life that comes to you through food. A prayerful attitude relaxes you, prepares your digestive system to assimilate fully the food you eat, and enables you to draw more prana from your food.

7.  When you are eating, simply EAT! Avoid distractions such as talking, reading, listening to the radio, or watching television. Conversation can create mental disturbances, and, at the least, it and other activities divert your attention from the awareness that is necessary to chew food properly and taste it fully. So when you talk or read while eating, your body must work harder to derive maximum benefit from the food. If you need to talk, make sure your conversation is gentle, pleasant, and loving.

8.  Make eating an act of meditation, of reverence for your body and your inner self. Be fully aware of what is occurring within your body. Visualize your digestive process and feel that the food is being converted into pranic energy for the sustenance of your body, mind, and spirit.

9.  If you overeat, accept yourself! You probably will overeat at times and that is natural. Learning to eat consciously happens gradually, so that there will be occasions when you forget or choose not to pay attention to your body's needs and instead listen to the mind's artificial demands.

    The most important thing at such times is to accept yourself and not create emotional tension and guilt about having eaten too much. Emotional reactions to eating will do more harm than the overeating itself. What's more, they will probably lead to more overeating, because they create tension in you.

    So if you overeat, don't worry about it. Learn from your experience; try to examine what led to your overeating, and correct the conditions for the next time.

In summary, for better overall health of body, mind, emotions, and spirit, eat consciously. Start by simplifying your diet, learning to become aware of the ways that different foods affect your energy and consciousness, and beginning to purify your system through more exercise and moderate fasting. (One day a week of fasting is very helpful, but even once a month is good.)

Always remember that balance and patience are the keys. Recognize and accept that it may take time to change ingrained habits and that diet and nutrition are only one of the eight pathways of the Kripalu Approach to health.

# Another Health Tool to Try

## Colon Cleansing

### Its History

Colonic cleansing in one form or another has a venerable history. Over 6,000 years ago, the earliest yogis experienced an automatic process they called *basti* occurring as their bodies were purified by their practices. They found that when they immersed themselves in water, spontaneous muscular contractions occurred that drew water into the colon to cleanse it. They later formalized the procedure as one of the cleansing techniques of yoga that are called *kriyas*.

People of other lands have developed methods of cleaning out the intestines through more mechanical means.

### Its Benefits

Many years of observing the experiences of hundreds of residents and visitors have led us to believe that some form of colonic cleansing is desirable at different stages on the path to greater health. That is because there is a factor in disease that yogis and ancient healers have known for thousands of years: much illness and disease, particularly chronic, is a result of a general toxemia (toxic blood).

Toxemia begins in the colon where uneliminated food wastes remain trapped and become bonded with mucus, forming an encrustation. Beneficial bacteria are destroyed as their environment is polluted and, as putrefaction sets in, toxic bacteria are released. The latter are absorbed into the bloodstream through the intestinal walls, are circulated in the body, and begin to cause disease and degeneration of healthy body tissues.

The colon, encrusted as it is, loses its elasticity and ability to undergo peristalsis, thereby further slowing down the elimination of wastes. The longer that waste products remain in the body, the more putrefaction and resulting toxic products are created. The toxins in turn cause further degeneration of muscle tone in the colon and a vicious circle is initiated.

What is the original cause of colon problems? There are many. Most experts believe that our present-day diet of over-refined, chemical-laden food and our habit of taking laxatives are major causative factors, along with the extreme tensions experienced in our fast-moving society. Whatever the cause, the results are tangible and experiential.

Many Americans suffer from some form of eliminative disorder, usually chronic constipation. The healthy body should have a bowel movement at least once or twice a day and, ideally, food should pass through the body within about twenty-four hours. Most people experience fewer bowel movements that that, and it may take up to seventy-two hours for the complete ingestion/elimination process.

Even if we are not suffering from any apparent digestive problems, it is estimated that most Americans carry up to five to ten pounds of encrusted, hardened feces lining their colons and inhibiting the body's ability to absorb fully the nutrients in food.

Enemas can help with the removal of material on the colon walls. The usual experience after an enema is a sense of well-being and greater vitality and health, even among those who are already evidencing good health.

## One Method of Colon Cleansing

An enema is a self-administered form of colon washing. Usually, it consists of suspending a special, flexible bag of water (or other liquid) two to three feet above the buttocks and allowing the liquid to flow gently into the body, in slow stages.

Simple enemas, if taken with skilled guidance, greatly reduce toxicity and facilitate elimination, which reduces constipation. Enemas are particularly helpful at the onset of colds or flu and can sometimes eliminate the toxicity that made one susceptible to the attack from germs or viruses. They are also excellent while fasting. (We would say indispensable on longer fasts.)

1. Obtain an enema bag (Most drug stores carry them, and the cost is minimal.) and an 18-inch catheter tube.

2. Find a suitable, quiet bathroom and toilet where you can remain undisturbed for thirty to forty-five minutes and where you can lie down comfortably.

3. Fill the enema bag with one to two quarts of warm to tepid water (body temperature) or other liquid (see below), and suspend it two to three feet above the ground. Allow the liquid to flow out from the bag for two or three seconds to remove any air bubbles.

4. Lubricate the nozzle and your anus with a little vegetable oil and assume a comfortable position. Various positions are possible, and the ultimate choice is personal. We recommend any of the following:

    (a) lying on your side with your knees slightly bent — first lying on the left side, then the back, then the right — and drawing your right knee up to your chest while retaining the water;

    (b) kneeling on all fours; or

    (c) lying on your back with hips raised by a small pillow or some towels.

    Assume whichever position feels most comfortable and facilitates the best flow. You may want to vary your position.

5. Insert the nozzle into your anus.

6. Gently controlling its flow with the clip on the hose of the enema bag, allow the liquid to trickle slowly into your colon. You will experience the desire to evacuate from time to time, but unless there is real pain or cramping, resist the urge as long as you can. Stopping the flow and massaging the colon will help eliminate the air pockets that can cause discomfort.

7. Ideally, work toward holding the liquid for a period of ten to twenty minutes (more or less, depending on the liquid). At first you may be able to hold only very little water for a very short period of time. With practice, you will be able to hold more and longer.

    After you hold and expel several small quantities, you may refill the bag. You will be able to hold more as you evacuate more waste. It is important to be gentle, yet firm with your body. Try not to evacuate as soon as you feel the urge, but avoid forcing or straining.

## What Liquid Should You Use?

1. Water (warm, not hot).

2. Lemon water (just a small quantity of freshly strained lemon juice added: perhaps three to four teaspoons per two quarts).

3. Weak chamomile tea or comfrey tea (helps eliminate mucus).

There are many other more or less exotic mixtures that can be used for specific purposes, but those should only be used at the advice and with the supervision of a holistic health specialist.

### CAUTION

Those with any kind of colon disease should first consult a specialist before attempting an enema.

Also, it is quite easy to become addicted to enemas as a substitute for laxatives or proper eating. Enemas are for occasional purification or crisis intervention and should not become habitual, as they may destroy muscle tone in the intestines or create other complications.

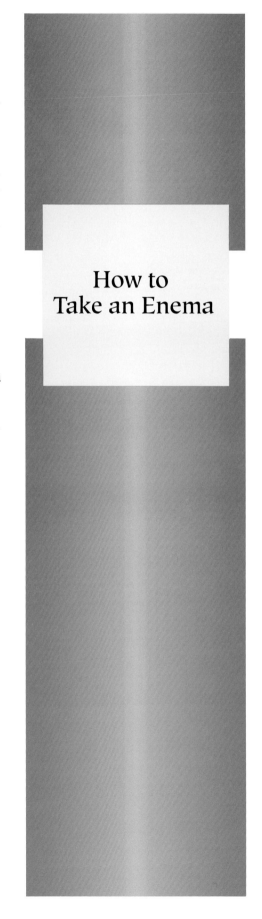

# How to
# Take an Enema

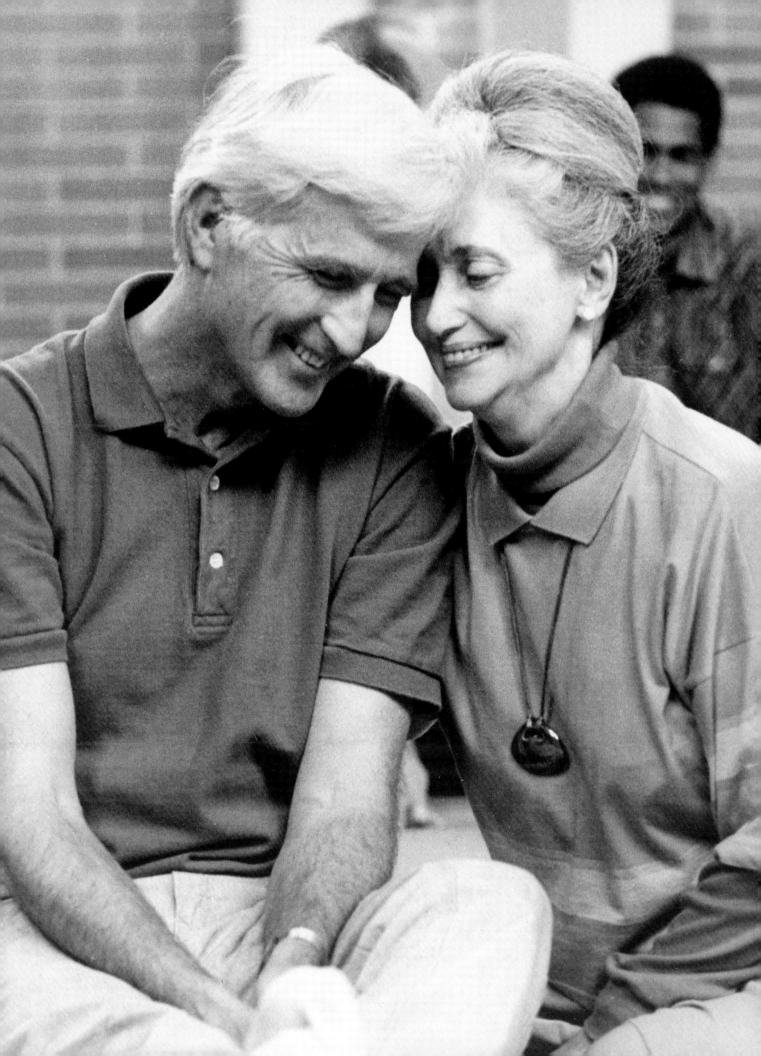

# The Sixth Pathway

mastering communication — with yourself and others

# The Importance of Communication

How many people do you communicate with in an average day? Probably dozens. Hundreds in a week, thousands in a year, and who knows how many in a lifetime. From the most casual and superficial interactions to the most intimate human relationships, our moments are filled with communications. They are the very lifeblood of our existence as social beings.

Our methods of communicating have evolved tremendously since the first ape man grunted to his neighbor. First the idea of language slowly evolved, then languages themselves, and then written forms, from primitive picture alphabets through cuneiform script to the present simplified letter alphabets of the West. It could well be said that the history of communication is the history of civilization.

The invention of printing in the fifteenth century made it possible for one person's ideas to influence many and catapulted mankind into a new phase of communications in which exchanges were no longer just interpersonal. In the last century we have seen an explosion of communication systems, from typewriter to tape recorder, from wireless to video to computer modem.

It seems that we are now awash in a sea of machines and our eyes and ears are bombarded day and night with messages. Where once communication was a seemingly simple phenomenon of one person talking or signaling to another, now we are all intercepting (willingly or unwillingly) millions of messages to and from everyone in society.

And our communication-bearing techniques and technologies have become increasingly sophisticated: more messages can be carried farther and faster to more people in more locations than ever before in history.

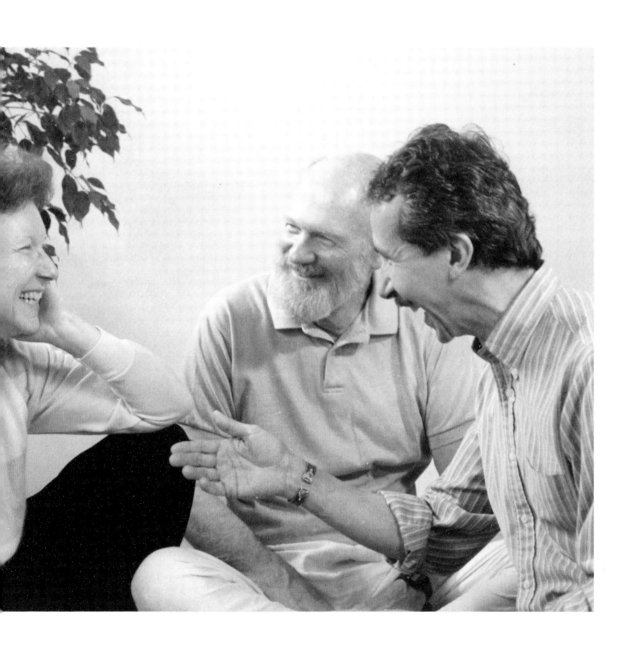

## More Is Not Necessarily Better

The question is, has the quality of our communications improved along with the quantity? Do we communicate on the person-to-person level better or only more and faster? Has the communications explosion helped us understand each other more deeply as human beings, or is the noise of our words deafening us so that it is increasingly difficult to hear each other?

And how has the growth of communication affected our consciousness? Have we become so skilled at exchanging messages regarding facts, opinions, and theories that we have overlooked the exchange of our feelings? Can we express feelings clearly? Do we know how to listen to another's expression?

There is no doubt that the efficiency of message delivery systems, such as books, film, television, and advertising, is at an all-time high. There is now a communications industry, with professional "communicators" and communications experts. There are degrees offered in communications. Yet we still find that true understanding between one individual and another is often blocked by communication problems. Marriages flounder and nations go to war because of breakdowns in communication.

Every interaction we have with another human being is a communication, with the potential to draw the two of us closer in love and understanding (and thus to participate in drawing all the people of the world closer) or to increase the distance between us.

What we think of as a simple transaction with a clerk in a store can make or break both our day and his or hers; interactions with loved ones and co-workers are even more intensely potent. Few experiences in life are as satisfying as feeling that we are truly understood by another human being, yet we still encounter difficulties.

What is it that blocks true communication between people? And how can we improve our communication skills so that we can overcome those blocks? What is the secret of good communication?

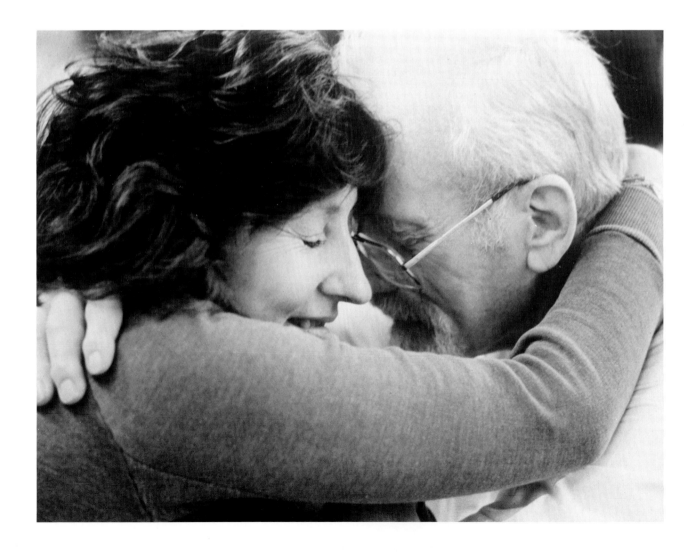

## Awareness

1. Write a few brief sentences using the words *communication* and *communicate* in as many different ways as you can, simply to illustrate their range of meanings.

2. Look over what you have written, and summarize briefly what these two words seem to mean for you.

3. See if you can think of any other meanings you may have missed and jot them down, too.

4. Reflect for a moment on how you feel when you hear the word *communication*. What associations does it bring up for you? What images? What emotions? Jot them down.

5. Complete the following sentences:

    (a) My communications with other people are usually…

    (b) I feel my ability to communicate with other people is…

    (c) When I have a good clear communication with someone, I feel ( emotionally and physically)…

    (d) When I am involved in a miscommunication of some kind I feel (emotionally and physically)…

    (e) When I am involved in a miscommunication with someone else, it is usually because…

    (f) I think most misunderstandings between people are caused by…

    (g) When I do have a clear, harmonious communication with another person, it is because…

    (h) I think I would be able to communicate better with other people if…

    (i) What I would like most to learn about communication is…

## Self-Discovery Experience

# 13

### How well do you communicate?

Before reading further, complete this Self-Discovery Experience to see where you stand and to gain an experiential basis for understanding the material in this chapter.

**Note**: Some questions are worded in a very similar way, yet are quite different in meaning. Be sure to answer exactly what is asked.

After reading each question, close your eyes and relax, allowing the answer to emerge in feelings and intuitions and writing it down without censoring.

## Acceptance and Adjustment

The Acceptance and Adjustment sections of this Self-Discovery Experience follow later in this chapter. Read the intervening material before completing them.

# Communications and Your Health

Have you ever stopped to consider the hidden messages behind some of our more common idiomatic expressions? Reflect for a moment on what these familiar phrases are saying:

"He's a real pain in the neck!" "I had to eat my words!" "I had to bite back what I was going to say." "I really cannot stomach that woman!" "I'll just have to shoulder the responsibility." "She is positively guilt ridden." "I swallowed my humiliation." "He certainly approaches life with a stiff upper lip."

There are many others. What they indicate is a close link between how we express ourselves and how we feel physically. They also demonstrate very clearly that when we are not able to express what we are feeling or interact harmoniously with others on the spoken level, there is a blockage in our flow of energy, a holding down or in of our prana.

Communication is the external expression of the energy of who we are. How we express ourselves, how that expression is received by others, and how we feel about our ability to communicate are key factors in our experience of health. Communication is particularly important in the holistic model of health, which looks at the well-being of the whole person and not just the physical body.

What do we mean, then, when we use the words *communication* and *communicate*? Probably your definition includes some of the following: to tell, to explain, to express an opinion, to convey facts, to make someone understand something, or simply to talk. All those meanings are correct, and yet they are incomplete if their underlying assumption is that communication always requires two people.

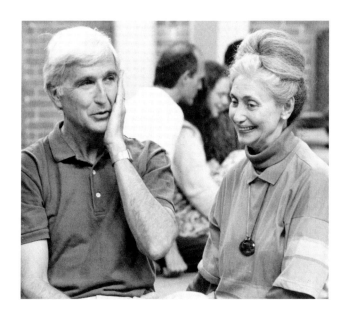

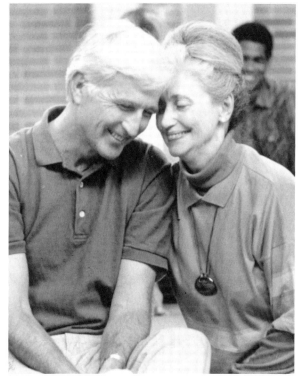

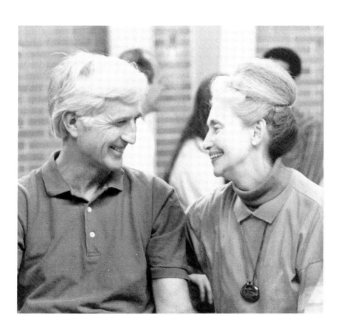

### First Learn to Communicate with Yourself

A basic dictionary definition of *communicate* is "to impart or exchange knowledge." Another definition given is "to make known," and that "making known" also happens within us. We must make our feelings known to ourselves on an inner level before we can begin to communicate them to others.

In the first section of this chapter, then, we will look at communication as an internal, as well as, and even prior to, an external process. Yogi Desai has said: "Until you learn to communicate with yourself, you cannot hope to communicate effectively with others." So we will look at communicating with ourselves as a first step to better communications with others.

There is a second possible misapprehension about the phenomenon of communication. It is that communication is an exchange: I communicate something to you and then you communicate something back to me. That view assumes that speaking is an active process requiring energy and listening is a passive process that doesn't take energy.

In the second section of the chapter we will look at a concept called "active listening," a type of listening that requires as much — if not more — energy and attention as speaking does. Until we can put as much energy and love into listening to others as we do into expressing our own points of view and feelings, we will not make others feel really heard, and true communication will not happen.

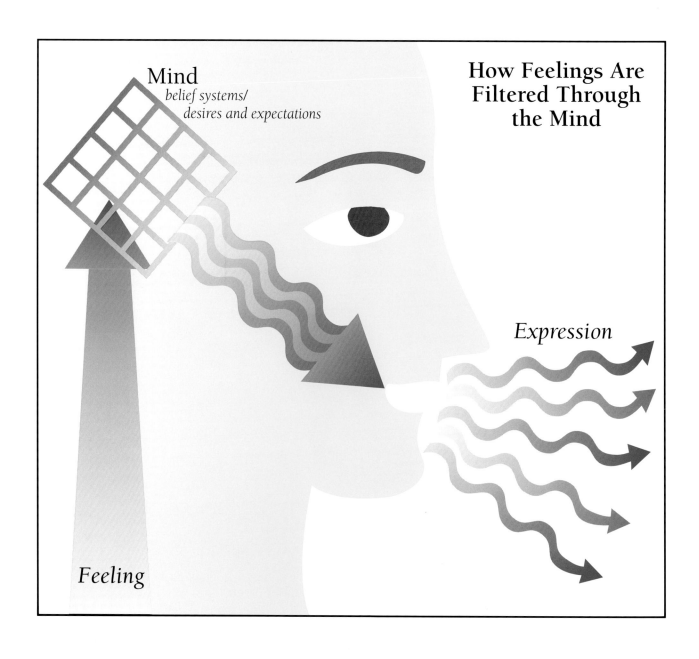

Mind
*belief systems/
desires and expectations*

How Feelings Are Filtered Through the Mind

*Expression*

*Feeling*

# Communication Skills I: Self-Expression

## You Don't Understand Me because I'm Afraid to Tell You Who I Am

Communication is a process that happens on two levels: the level of experience and the level of expression. The first level concerns our communication with ourselves; the second, our communication with others. Both are equally important. Our feelings are at the core of our experience of life; our communication with others is essential for our survival in the world and for our sense of connection with fellow human beings.

Miscommunication or poor communication with others is a common experience. It is behind most of our difficulties with other people. Miscommunication with ourselves (our lack of ability to understand what is really going on inside us) is often at the root of any tension or discomfort we may feel.

Even if we feel that we already communicate well with those around us, a deeper understanding of our inner communication system will still yield benefits in the form of a more harmonious, flowing, and loving life.

## The Process of Expressing

How do the internal and external communication problems arise? In our personal internal communications network, there is a frequently overlooked process that is responsible for most communication problems. It is the process that happens to our feelings between the time we sense them and the time we express them.

Most of us are awkward in expressing our feelings at one time or another. The reason is that when we prepare to express ourselves, a complex chain of events takes place inside us, occurring so fast that we are usually not conscious of it. That chain of inner events often results in a distortion of the original feeling that was our authentic experience.

It is difficult to express feelings, which are nonverbal and nonconceptual, in the form of language, which must necessarily work through words and concepts. To that difficulty we add another of trying to express something that we ourselves do not really understand, because we have lost touch with the original, basic feeling that motivated us to speak.

So what we are conscious of wanting to express is often quite different from what we originally felt. And because our bodies manifest the effects of our feelings, when what we eventually try to express is something different from the original feeling, a split occurs between body and mind, feeling and expression.

That split results in physical tension and emotional frustration at our inability to express what we are experiencing. It leads to feelings of lack of love because we feel that the person listening does not understand what we are trying to say. Really it is we who do not know what we are trying to say, because we no longer know what it is we are feeling. Yet we are not aware that we do not know; we believe we are simply unable to express what we feel.

## Bridging the Gap between Feeling and Expression

We need somehow to bridge the gap between feeling and expression. To do that we must understand the unconscious internal process that distorts the feelings we have before we can recognize them consciously and work at expressing them.

The tools we use to integrate experiences into our lives are our minds. The role of the mind is to note, consciously and objectively, what we are feeling in our bodies, interpret what that means in terms of our need to interact with the outside world, and then provide us with words or other means of communication to carry out that interaction.

## The Mind as a Distorting Filter

Unfortunately, that mental process has become distorted. The original cause of the distortion is fear, but we do not recognize it as that because it has grown habitual. Now our minds are no longer able to perceive our feelings objectively and clearly.

Over the years the mind has acquired the qualities of a filter, so that it transmits only a part of the light of our feelings. Or we could compare the mind to a distorting lens that bends the rays of light of our feelings as they pass through and makes them unrecognizable.

The mind's distorting lens or filter is composed of two major elements: our belief systems formed in response to the mind's perceptions of past events and our desires and expectations for the future.

We want very much to control the present and the future, so that they turn out differently from our memories of unsuccessful past experiences. So we are constantly, albeit unconsciously, trying to use the present to right unremembered wrongs of the past.

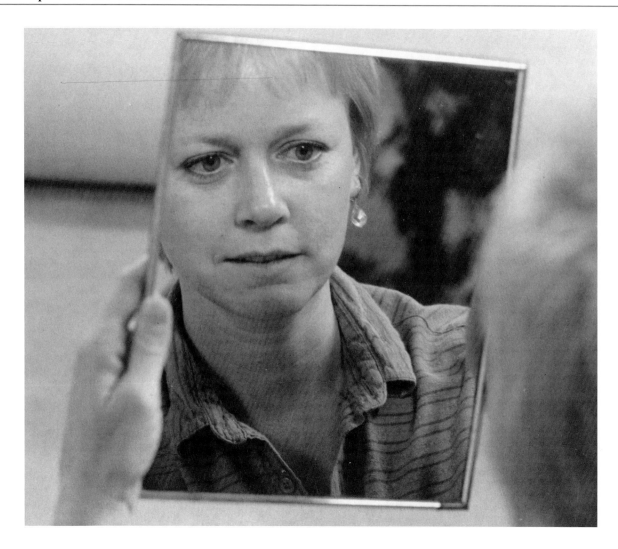

For our mind-body complex, the past is an unfinished gestalt, an incomplete circle we are trying to complete. So each communication in the present is an unconscious attempt to achieve a desired communication we didn't achieve in the past.

## "When I Was a Child, I Spake as a Child . . ."

As small children, we naturally and spontaneously expressed our feelings as they arose. We had no verbal ability, so we did not try to translate them into words. If you watch small children, you will see that. Joy, anger, pain, and hunger are all expressed spontaneously through the body, with laughter, shouts, or tears, and pass quickly and are forgotten. There is no inhibition or holding back.

As we grew older we began to find, to our shocked surprise, that some of those spontaneous expressions of feeling were no longer acceptable; they were considered childish, negative, or inappropriate to mature, civilized human beings.

We learned it was "bad" to express anger by striking or shouting. We were told not to cry, because only babies (or girls) cry. We were made to control our hunger until it was time to eat or to ask for food rather than cry for it.

Because of our need for approval, which is one of the deepest of human needs, we learned to fear the expression of our feelings, to inhibit and mask them, and even to feel guilty about having them at all.

## From Mask to Mask

As we learned to express ourselves through language, we struggled to find words that would express our feelings in a way that was acceptable to the powerful adults in our lives: our parents and teachers. We began to wear masks, in order to disguise our true feelings from others and protect ourselves from criticism and disapproval.

Gradually we forgot that we were wearing a mask. The internal process of fear and denial of our true feelings happened so fast that we became unaware of it. It passed into our personality as a mechanical, habitual inner process, and we became distant from ourselves, living once-removed from our real experience.

But one denial and removal gradually necessitated another, and then another. It is like lying: one lie requires another to cover it up, then another to cover up the second one, and so on. We were constantly putting on a new mask to cover up the old, whenever we feared that the old one had become unacceptable.

## Believing Our Own Pretense

So, in order to be acceptable to others and gain their approval, we pretended to be different from our true selves. And we ended up believing our pretense, so that we could make sense of our inner universe.

The phenomenon of believing our own pretense is illustrated by a psychological theory called "cognitive dissonance." It states that when we hold two contradictory cognitions, or perceptions, about our environment, our subconscious mind distorts one of those perceptions in order to eliminate the mental dissonance (the disharmony) that results from trying to encompass both.

That means that our drive for inner consistency is so powerful that the mind spontaneously and unconsciously lies to itself in order to produce agreement between two discordant elements. And that is what happens in our communication system.

If our underlying beliefs are that "If I want to be accepted, I must be a good person" and "A good person is not supposed to feel angry," then our mental syllogism concludes: "So, I am not angry." The intermediate step of "I may experience anger, but I will not show it" is often unconsciously omitted.

Ironically enough, we begin our self-deception out of a fear of being rejected, and we end up experiencing rejection anyway, not because we are angry but because we are not expressing our real feelings. We are not being real, and other people are able to feel that on a subtle level, even if they don't interpret the feeling consciously.

So we go around wearing masks — rejecting ourselves and rejecting each other — all because we have habitually allowed our fear of rejection, which may have been an illusion in the first place, to distort who we are and who we say we are.

We are thus trapped in a vicious circle, the results of which are profound. Not only are we unable to communicate clearly with others, but we have lost the ability to communicate clearly with ourselves. The fact is that most of us no longer know what it is we are feeling. We no longer know who we really are. The gap between our feeling, our thinking, and our action is so wide that we are like different people trapped in the same body.

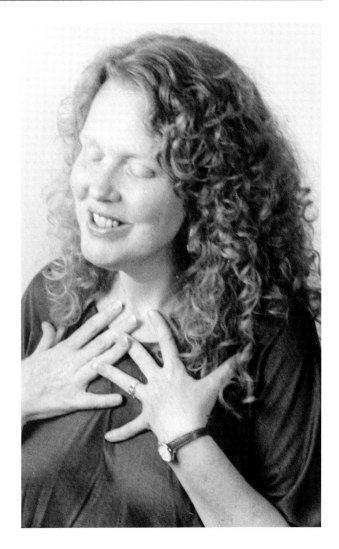

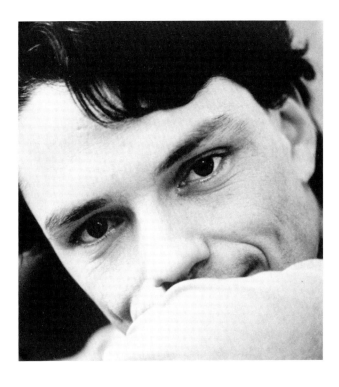

## Accepting Our Feelings as They Are

How do we begin to bridge that gap? First, by observing ourselves closely in order to see where we deny our original feeling out of fear, how we distort it, and what the result of that distortion is. We must bring the whole unconscious, mechanical process under the spotlight of our awareness.

Then, in order to be able to view our feelings objectively and with clarity, we must be willing to let go of our fear, both of others' rejection and of self-rejection. We must begin to accept our feelings just as they are.

That does not mean we have to express all our feelings — that is a different matter — but we do need to recognize, without guilt, that whatever our feeling is in a given situation, is a perfectly natural, human response. Only when we are clear about what we are feeling and have accepted it, can we communicate it to another.

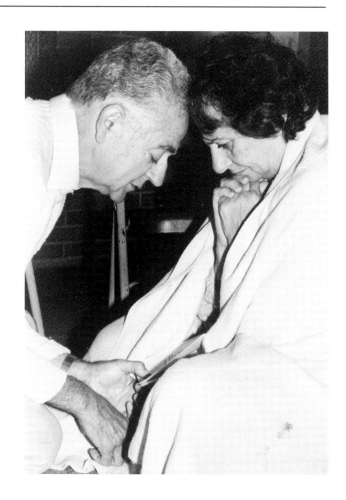

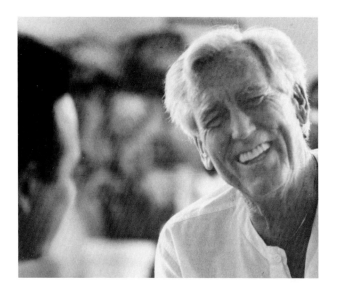

## STOP!

How aware are you of your body messages right now? How are you feeling? Is there tension, stiffness, or tiredness in any part of your body? Do you need to get up and stretch? Take some deep breaths? Relax your shoulders? Rest your eyes? Rest your mind? Close your eyes for a minute and take some long, slow, deep breaths to enable you to get in touch with your experience. Then respond to what your body is asking you to do.

## Acceptance

Review the answers to the questions in the Awareness section (p. 167). Read them as if they were written by someone else and you were being asked to evaluate them. As a detached observer, look for and write down the following:

6.  Patterns that you see in your communications that may lead to communication problems.

7.  Your strengths in communicating with others.

8.  Your greatest areas of weakness. For example: Do you feel easily frustrated when you are not understood? Do you feel inadequate and unable to express yourself in certain situations? Are you at ease in communicating facts, figures, and opinions, but insecure in talking about your emotions and feelings?

9.  Your blind spots in communications. Do you tend to blame others for communication difficulties or to retreat into shyness to avoid situations?

10. Any other observations that occur to you that may be helpful.

Be sure to maintain an objectivity about your observations. Accept that it seems to be the human condition to have difficulty in expressing feelings, so if you experience that difficulty, it simply shows that you are human. Remember also that language is, at best, simply an approximation of what is going on inside us.

## Adjustment

11. Write down several specific areas of your communication skills that you would like to work on improving.

12. As you go through the rest of this chapter, make notes as you encounter further areas you'd like to work on.

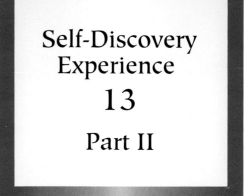

# Self-Discovery Experience 13
## Part II

**How well do you communicate?**

Once we have understood and accepted that the first step in good external communications is to have good internal communications, the question becomes "How can I learn to understand my inner communications more clearly?"

On the following pages are two techniques. The first is a form of introspection that follows the "three-A" format (Awareness, Acceptance, Adjustment). It outlines questions you can ask yourself to get clear about your part in a specific situation of miscommunication or conflict. Often, if you are able to formulate the right questions, you will find the seeds of the answers in the questions themselves.

The second technique is to help clarify the feelings, awarenesses, and observations that come up on a daily basis. It takes the form of a written communications journal with a special format to help you gain insights by seeing patterns in what you record.

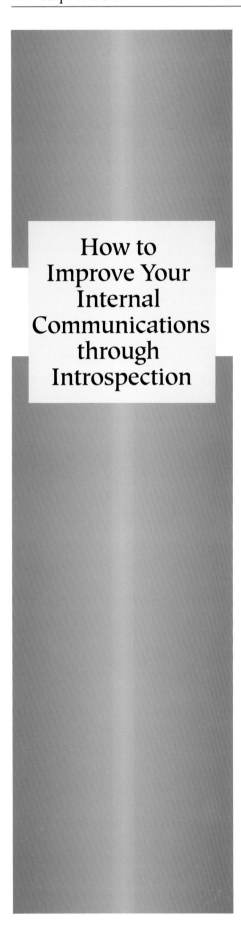

## How to Improve Your Internal Communications through Introspection

Whenever you have a conflict with someone, examine the situation carefully in an honest and open way, at a time when you are no longer feeling any of the strong emotions that were present when you were in the situation.

The following exercise, which facilitates that examination, has helped many people resolve conflicts with others and within themselves. Using this method will increase your understanding, enhance your inner harmony, and make your communication with those around you more effective.

Begin by relaxing your body and mind as you close your eyes and take a few long deep breaths.

Choose a situation or conflict you would like to understand more clearly and use for your growth. Resolve to seek the lesson for you in that situation in an honest and open manner.

Write down your answers to the following questions and statements as clearly and objectively as you can:

1. Describe what happened.
2. Ask "What did I. . . think?"
   feel?"
   do?"
   say?"
3. Now, as honestly and completely as you can, put yourself in the other person's place. Ask "What did he/she . . . think?"
   feel?"
   do?"
   say?"
4. Ask "What did I want from the situation?" Again putting yourself in the other person's place, ask "What did he/she want?"
5. In every situation of conflict, there is some underlying fear on both sides. Ask yourself: "What were the fears in this situation?" "What was I afraid of deep down?" "What was he/she afraid would or would not happen?"
6. Taking all the above into consideration, ask "What was the effect of my action(s). . . on the other person?"
   . . . on me?"
7. Finally, ask "How would I want to do it differently next time?"
8. Reread your answers to the above questions. Reflect on what you have learned about the ways in which you contributed to the conflict you have dealt with. Be aware of the fact that neither you nor the other person was to blame, but that you both had a point of view and feelings that would not allow you to hear each other objectively.
9. Now that you have explored some of the feelings on both sides, experience the clarity that comes from objective and open internal communication. That kind of open communication with yourself leads to clear communication with others. You can use this exercise in many different situations situations to increase your awareness of your internal and external communication.

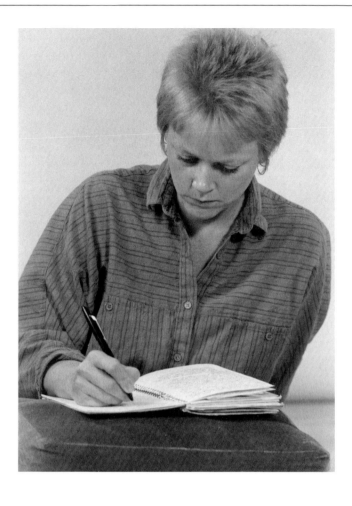

# How to Use a Journal to Improve Your Internal Communications

Writing in a special journal is another way for you to improve your internal process of communication. There are two ways the journal will work for you.

The first is getting in touch with your inner imagery as a way to uncover the deeper layers of your experience that are often buried under everyday concerns. Inner imagery flows when you put yourself in a meditative state and consciously allow the mind to relax.

In all the exercises below you will be able to record your imagery in your journal as you experience it in the moment. It is important to remember that imagery does not mean strictly mental pictures. It also includes feelings, sounds, situations, or even smells that come to your inner awareness.

Holding an inner dialogue is another way for you to let the different parts of yourself become more conscious. The conversation actually takes the form of a written dialogue in which you become both speakers.

The dialogue technique is profoundly effective because it allows you to voice clearly both sides of any conflicting situation arising in your life, whereas normally you might suppress one side or perhaps not even be aware of its existence.

You may find yourself saying things in your dialogue that you didn't know you felt. You may encounter within you a surprising wisdom that will move you toward a healing acceptance, understanding, and reconciliation of the opposing elements in the conflicts you experience.

# A Suggested Way of Working in Your Journal

1. Keep a daily record of any situations that arise that seem to have a special emotional, mental, or spiritual significance. It may be an interaction with someone you work closely with, that allows you to see something in your relationship you've never seen before. You may have a deep experience doing a new posture, or a breakthrough in your job. Or you may wake up one morning with an unusual feeling about yourself.

   This daily record will give you material to work with when you want to get a perspective on your life by self-reflection in the form of journal writing.

2. Schedule a time during the week when you can review the events recorded in your daily record. Sit in a relaxed position and ask yourself the question "What does each of the events I've recorded tell me about myself — about my emotions, my physical body, my mind and the way it works, and my spiritual growth?"

3. Select an event or situation in which your feelings seem unclear or unfinished. Sit with that situation for a moment, with your eyes closed, and enter into a quiet, meditative state. Allow the thoughts about the situation to dissolve and simply feel the feelings involved.

   That is the stage in which your own inner images will rise to the surface. Simply record the images as they come, without editing or judging. After listing the images, reread the list and ask "What do these images tell me about myself?"

   Images are your own inner wisdom speaking to you in another language — a language that is closer to your feelings as you actually experience them, rather than as you think about them. Ask "What are these images telling me about myself that I am not hearing in any other way?"

   Write a brief statement about the situation, saying what you imagine the images are communicating about your inner feelings, needs, or thoughts.

4. You are now ready to enter into a dialogue about the situation. As you bring your inner voices into your awareness, you may notice that you feel two (or more) seemingly opposite pulls on your energy because of conflicting feelings and images you hold of yourself. The technique of an internal conversation allows you to explore very deeply the apparently conflicting elements within you, because you concentrate on identifying the opposing messages you give yourself.

In order to facilitate this process for the first few times, you may need to sit with your eyes closed for a moment to get in touch with your feelings before writing.

Some examples of opposing internal voices that might be the two parties in your dialogue are:

- the weak you and the strong you;
- the you that you think is a success and the you that you think is a failure;
- the you who wants to grow and the you who feels safer remaining with things that are known;
- the closed, resistant part of you and the open, accepting part of you;
- your mind and your body;
- the fat you and the skinny you;
- the part of you that wants control and the part of you that wants to let go;
- the part of you that wants to be independent and alone, and the part of you that wants to be accepted by others;
- the part of you that wants to know who you are and the part of you that is afraid to know;
- the part of you that is feminine and the part that is masculine;
- the part of your job you enjoy and the part you don't;
- the part of you that feels vulnerable and resists change and the part that is fearless and wants to try new experiences.

5. Accept yourself as you are. By allowing yourself the time to hear the conversations that constantly go on in your life, you have begun the process of accepting yourself honestly, as you are.

   As you accept more and more of the person you find that you are, you open the door to understanding yourself and your needs. Personal growth is the natural outcome of accepting, understanding, and being ready to change the things you see in your life that hold you back from being yourself.

   You can see that the enumeration of possible internal conversations could go on endlessly. The list above is just to give you a general idea of some areas where you might begin to bring into conscious awareness the people, experiences, feelings, fears, pleasures, and growths that make up the events of your life.

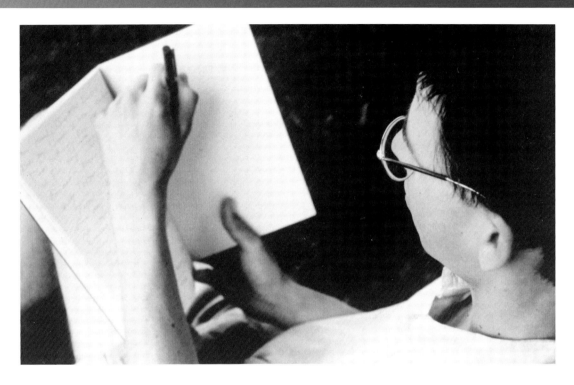

You will discover that both parts or sides of you that you identify in your dialogue are acceptable and natural; there is no need to experience them as conflicting but rather as complementary. Once you acknowledge them clearly, the need to negate one will drop away. They can both coexist harmoniously, even if you must, of necessity, choose to act upon only one.

To hold an inner dialogue with yourself, go through the following steps:

(a) Sit quietly for a moment and recall a situation where you experienced some inner conflict or indecision. Identify what seem to be the two (or several) voices in the conflict, using the preceding list for guidance.

(b) Allow one voice to begin to speak about the situation in words or feelings. Listen carefully and, as the words become clear, write down what that voice is saying. It is better not to think too much about the process, as that may inhibit your experience; just allow the feelings to be expressed in words.

(c) Allow the other voice to respond to what the first voice said. Again let it come from your feelings without too much thinking. Let whatever words seem to express the feelings come, even if they seem strange to your rational mind — even if your first reaction is "That isn't me; that isn't how I think!"

(d) Allow the dialogue to continue, alternating the voices as long as it seems necessary for you to clarify the inner process that is going on. You will find that after a certain time, you will feel complete.

(e) Go back over what you have written and see what you can learn from it.

(f) Finally, turn inward to your higher self, your inner guide, and ask for guidance in interpreting and implementing what you have seen in yourself. That is best done through meditation: sitting quietly, relaxing consciously, and allowing the answers to flow to you from the deep source of intuitive knowledge that becomes available to you at such times.

Every enlightened master describes our human nature as being both loving and able to receive love. Your true self is just that, so listening to yourself will provide you with the highest, most loving guidance possible.

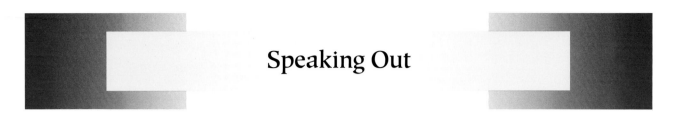

# Speaking Out

Once our internal communications have greater clarity, we are in a position to communicate more clearly with others. But before we begin to communicate with those whom we experience as outside us, there are two life attitudes or ways of viewing the world that need to be cultivated, for they seem to be prerequisites to clear communication of any kind.

The first concerns self-responsibility: It is recognizing that you alone are the creator of your life experience, that no one else causes you to feel what you feel in response to a given situation. The second prerequisite attitude is seeing every situation that happens to you that you define as difficult as a perfect opportunity to learn more about yourself and to grow in understanding, patience, tolerance, and love.

If you approach communication with those two attitudes, then the aim of your communications will no longer be to change others, or to assign responsibility to them for creating difficulties in your life, but simply to share yourself with them, and your communication problems will begin to dissolve.

More help for clear communication is provided by the following essay in which Yogi Desai outlines seven key steps in communicating our feelings more clearly. The guidelines he gives can improve the quality of your communications. Each time you find yourself involved in any kind of miscommunication or misunderstanding, review the guidelines.

Using them as a checklist will help you to see where the miscommunication originated, how it has been perpetuated, and what you can do, in very specific ways, to right the situation. The more you work with them, the more you will internalize them until effortless communications begin to flow naturally through you.

# Seven Steps to Clearer Communication with Others

### by Yogi Amrit Desai

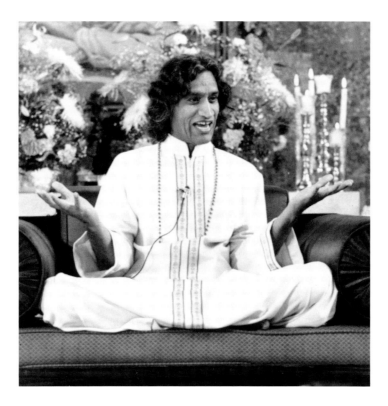

1. Examine the basic life attitudes that underlie your feelings. When you understand at a deep level that your happiness lies, not in how much you can change the world by getting others to respond to you in the way you'd like, but in changing the world inside you, then you will begin to change your perspective on life and your mind will become clear and objective.

   Those who have the greatest lack of objectivity are people who see the world as the source of their problems in miscommunication and think that they themselves are always right. They are always trying to change other people and external conditions to solve their problems rather then working on themselves.

2. Accept responsibility for your part in any misunderstanding. If you are involved in a misunderstanding with another person, stop and ask yourself the question "Have I given enough time and understanding to the issue involved to ensure that I am fair and objective?" Then ask, "Have I chosen appropriate words and considerate language to communicate my feelings clearly?"

   If you learn only that much, you will create a unique capacity to express yourself honestly and clearly. Whether the other people understand or not is ultimately beyond your control. You can help them only so far. Communicating objectively with others, without blaming them, is of greatest importance.

3. Put yourself in the other's place. Open your heart. Ask yourself: "Am I being sensitive to how he or she is feeling right now? Is my heart open?" If you can be as attuned to the other person's feelings as you are to your own, you will be able to express what you are feeling in a sensitive way and to choose the correct moment to express yourself.

   Even if you express what you feel with proper words, clear communication will not result if you choose the wrong moment to attempt it. The right moment is when you are objective and open to admitting your own responsibility in the conflict. Only then can you explain to the other where the misunderstanding arose in a kind and loving manner along with your carefully chosen words.

4. Become aware of what you want or expect from the other. Always ask, "What do I want from this person?" If you say what you imagine will make another person accept you, you will only be speaking the language

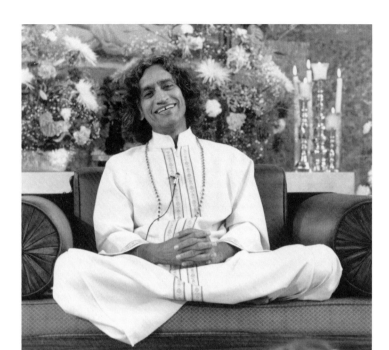

of fear. What you actually want will invariably color both the words you choose and your body language. Miscommunication is frequently a clash between two people trying to guard their security systems. If you understand what other people need for their security and give them that, as a way of loving them, you will have conquered many miscommunication problems. Also, if you feel secure in communicating with other people, you create the same security for them.

5. Balance self-responsibility with patience and self-acceptance. As your consciousness begins to awaken and you develop greater objectivity, you will be unable to place blame for your miscommunications totally on other people. You will see that you have more responsibility than you thought for your conflicts. And then you may begin to place all the blame on yourself for the problems around you and experience guilt, self-hatred, or an inferiority/superiority complex.

At that point it may seem that you have more problems than before your consciousness began to awaken, but that is not so: You are simply more aware of what is happening. This is why accepting the responsibility for your communications needs to be balanced with self-acceptance, patience, and self-love. And as you see more, through your increased awareness, you will also begin to see your own need for self-acceptance more clearly.

6. Develop a compassionate objectivity. When you develop objectivity you see the inside and outside of yourself as you really are without blame or guilt.

That allows you to communicate with yourself and see your problems clearly. Compassionate objectivity is essential for moving from self-blame to self-acceptance.

With a compassionate objectivity, you can also help others transcend their problems by offering new perspectives that only a loving objectivity allows. Psychological techniques may be able to bring people out of their difficulties, but they cannot give a perspective that will sustain people in that condition long enough to transcend the problem. Therefore they will soon become victims of similar problems again.

7. Recognize that the ultimate benefit of good communication is the realization of who you really are. With inner communication comes realization. You develop the capacity to become clear with yourself when you learn from experience that what you perceive as your problems actually lie within you and, therefore, you are the only one who can remove them.

A realization of that nature cannot come at a purely mental level. It can only happen experientially, at the heart level. You may hear certain things explained over and over again, but only when you have heard them experientially, through the heart, will you realize the implication of what is said and be able to practice it. You will be able to tell whether you have truly communicated with yourself by the change that each new realization brings to your life.

# How to Make Your Speech More Powerful . . .

**. . . Or: "I guess I'd really, sort of, like to, you know, learn to, er, speak, kind of, more clearly."**

There are many small expressions and interjections in our everyday speech that weaken it and result in our not being understood clearly, or even listened to by others. Those little words have become so habitual that we usually are not aware of the frequency with which we use them.

Even if we are aware, we may not realize the great effect they have, not only on how we communicate with others, but also on how others perceive us and how we perceive ourselves. Speech that is full of those words is tiresome to listen to and so ineffectual that people actually do not hear or do not believe what we are trying to say.

We call those small words and phrases *qualifiers* and *nullifiers*. They came into our speech at some time in the past when we felt insecure about what we were saying, or when we felt unable or unwilling, for some reason, to take full responsibility for our statements. Perhaps it started when we were young and we felt afraid that our feelings were not appropriate or would be criticized.

In any case, the words entered our vocabulary and became habitual as their use was reinforced by the fact that other people used them habitually also. But there is a paradox here. Originally, we used the phrases out of insecurity. Now they actually perpetuate our insecurity because we sense that they make our communication unclear.

Our thoughts and words affect how we feel about ourselves, even if we are not always aware of that at the conscious level. Changing our speech patterns can have a profound effect on how we experience life.

As you read the following examples of unclear speech and the suggested versions that follow each, say them aloud and be conscious of how you experience yourself differently. Then choose some examples of your own to practice with.

## Qualifiers

Qualifiers are myriad little words we unconsciously weave into our speech. They have no real meaning or function in themselves; they may seem to have a purpose, but usually they simply water down our speech, making it weak and indecisive.

For example:

"I guess I *really* don't want to do what you suggest."

Substitute: "I prefer not to do what you suggest."

"It's *sort of* hard to say, *you know*, who is right."

Substitute: "I find it hard to say who is right."

"*Well,* I feel *kind of, you know* . . . upset."

Substitute: "Right now I'm feeling upset."

"It's *kind of* a touchy subject."

Substitute: "For me this is a difficult subject."

"I *just* want to let you know that . . ."

Substitute: "I want to let you know that . . ."

"*Maybe* we could talk about it some other time."

Substitute: "Could we please talk about it some other time?"

"It's, *like,* difficult to answer. *I mean* . . ."

Substitute: "I find that difficult to answer."

In each case you will have observed that the second sentence feels more decisive, clear, and direct. The speaker is really taking responsibility, without equivocation, for what he or she is saying. In the first sentence, the speaker is obviously ill at ease with what he or she is saying, like a politician who makes a statement and then says quickly, "Don't quote me on that."

When we use qualifiers, we are indecisive. We want to say something, yet at the same time we don't want to because of the imagined consequences. Or more likely we were at one time afraid and now we have more confidence, but such words and phrases have become a deeply entrenched habit.

Teenagers and young people in particular tend to use qualifiers, because they are going through the insecurity of moving into the adult world where standards are different. Quite possibly we picked up the habit at that time in our lives.

The solution is to drop these extras phrases and say exactly what we feel. If we wish to soften our speech, it is better to do so by varying our tone of voice or simply by admitting that we are unsure of what we are about to say.

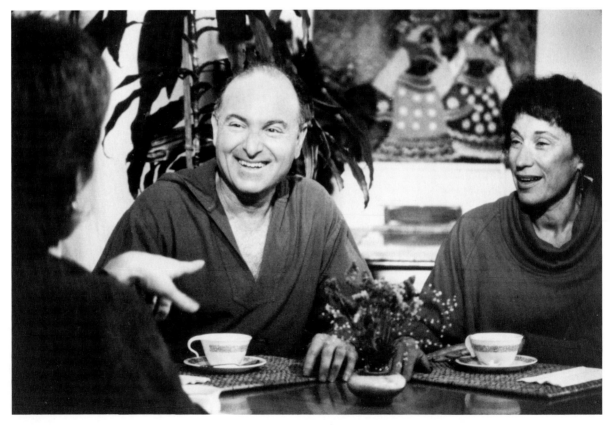

There is no shame in saying "I find it hard to express my feelings;" "I'm not sure of what I am about to say;" "I don't like to admit this because I feel vulnerable and weak;" or "I don't like to be wrong, so I am afraid to say this."

## Nullifiers

Nullifiers are words and phrases that tend to negate what we are saying or feeling and to fix permanently in time our concepts of ourselves and others, thus removing all possibility of change. They are very subtle and insidious ways in which we prevent ourselves from owning our feelings and communicating clearly.

Again, as you read aloud both versions of the sentences below, notice how there is a subtle difference in feeling from one to the other.

1. Change *but* to *and*.

   This admits the possibility of two parallel feelings existing in us at the same time, without any conflict or negation.

   Example: "I really love you, but sometimes I get angry at you."

   Instead say: "I really love you and . . ."

2. Change *I know* to *I imagine*.

   This gives the other person a chance to explain and not feel judged or defined.

   Example: "I know you're going to be angry with me."

   Instead say: "I imagine you may be angry with me; of course I may be wrong."

3. Change *I can't* to *I prefer not to*.

   This owns responsibility for the attitude expressed, and thus retains the power to change.

   Example: "I can't talk to you right now."

   Instead say: "I prefer not to talk to you right now."

4. Change *I have to* to *I choose to*.

   This is another opportunity to assume responsibility. It also avoids the feeling of resentment.

   Example: "I have to go on a diet because I have high blood pressure."

   Instead say: "I choose to eat in a new way for the sake of my health."

5. Change *I should* to *I could*.

   This again takes responsibility back from imaginary outside sources and owns the feeling.

   Example: "I should (ought to) get up early and go jogging."

   Instead say: "I could get up early and go jogging." (Then choose to do it or not.)

6. Change *I don't know* to *I can find out*.

   Instead of closing off all further possibilities, saying "I can find out" opens up new opportu-

nities to grow, feel good, and help others.

Example: "I don't know what to do."

Instead say: "I can find out what to do."

7. Change *always/never* to an appropriate statement that is less restricted.

   These two words are another example of limiting and permanently defining a person or a feeling. They can either be dropped altogether or replaced by phrases such as *sometimes*, *occasionally*, or *until now*.

   Example: "I always forget my wife's birthday."

   Instead say: "I have forgotten my wife's birthday until now, and this time I will remember."

   Example: "I never get to a meeting on time."

   Instead say: "Until now I haven't been able to get to a meeting on time. And I can change."

Improving your communication skills will have a profound impact on your whole sense of well-being and progress toward holistic health. You will find yourself feeling consistently both a greater relaxation and greater energy, because your prana will be flowing more freely as a result of your ability to express yourself in a clearer way.

As you learn to say what you want to say in a loving manner, you will feel greater freedom in your interactions with others, because you will feel confident in your ability to speak without hurting or antagonizing them. You will find that you experience a great sense of satisfaction when you conduct clearly a communication that in the past would have left you feeling tense, frustrated, angry, or depressed.

You will also experience others being more open to you, in a most surprising way, as they gain confidence in your openness and lack of desire to defend yourself or to manipulate them. Your ability and willingness to be real about your less noble feelings will open others' hearts to you, especially as you become able to express yourself with both honesty and gentleness.

True communication is more than just skill with words. It is the result of a gentle and open heart that knows no other way to express itself than honestly and lovingly.

# Communication Skills II: Active Listening

## "You Know I Can't Hear You When My Mind Is Running."

Another often neglected part of good communication is listening. We all value a good listener. We feel heard, understood, sympathized with, and loved, when someone really listens to us without argument or judgement. Much of the therapeutic benefit of talking to a good listener, whether psychiatrist, clergyman, or friend, is from the experience of being able to express freely what is bottled up inside without fear of the consequences.

Very often, we cannot express our feelings to those closest to us, and about whom we feel what we feel, because we are afraid of their reactions. We fear hurt; we fear judgement; we fear criticism; we fear misunderstanding and misinterpretation; we fear being rationalized out of our feelings; we fear being wrong; and we fear, most of all, being overwhelmed and negated. So we either close down or seek an uninvolved and objective third party to whom we can complain.

Yet, how often are we able to provide for others that open, nonjudgmental listening ear that we ourselves appreciate and need so much? How often do we start out by listening, only to jump in with our reactions, retorts, defenses, and justifications? How often are we able to hear someone out, without comment, simply allowing them to express all that they are feeling?

Even if we do remain silent, what is happening in our minds? Are we refuting them mentally at every step, lining up our arguments in response? ("That's simply not true! That's so unfair. I can't let him get away with that.") Are we judging them mentally ("Oh, she always gets so emotional.")?

What seems to happen to most of us is that we are so busy reacting that we cannot hear the other person properly. Even if we give the appearance of listening, our energies are all directed inward to our own inner dialogues. And usually our eyes, if not our whole body language, reveal that.

We've all experienced that feeling of "He/She is not with me — not really listening." There's a glazed look in the eyes and a restlessness in the body. Even if the person remains still, we sense in them a desire to move and fear that, at any minute, they may look at their watch, spring to their feet, or interrupt us.

True listeners, in contrast, exude deep receptivity, a patience and endless willingness to be with us and let us express ourselves. Their eyes are like deep, still pools, inviting us to plunge in. Their body language is saying "I am here for you as long as you need me. I am not here to refute you or negate you, but simply to hear you and receive you."

Such people are rare. Even those who have made a profession of listening may not always have that quality; their listening sometimes has an air of abstraction or practiced patience. Learning to truly listen shows a willingness to learn to be more loving, which also is an art that must be learned.

Knowing from experience what a great and loving gift true listening is, how can we learn to offer that gift to others? The secret sounds deceptively simple: Truly listening to others requires a degree of selflessness; it requires that we be able to put aside our needs and concerns for a period of time and simply be a mirror, in wordless empathy, allowing the other to see him- or herself more clearly.

Silent or what we call "active" listening allows the other person to hear his or her own words and feelings, rather than our responses. It is extremely difficult for most of us because we are so used to the responsive or reactive model of communication where speakers alternate, as in the following:

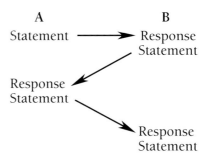

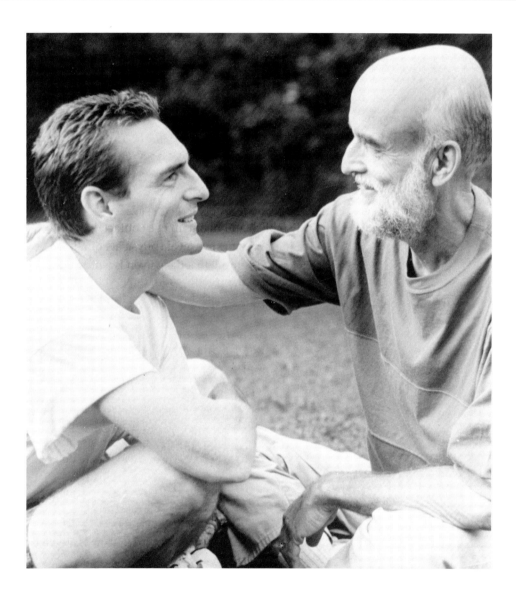

Communication in that model, is like a tennis game — and usually a very competitive one. Active listening, on the other hand, allows one player to keep on hitting, while the other simply receives the balls and lays them out in a row so that they can be seen clearly by both parties.

Mastering the art of active listening is one of the most rewarding things one can do in life. Experiencing our own openness is a reward in itself; it feels wonderful to lay aside our personal concerns for a moment and just be there for another person.

The second reward is the depth and honesty of the other person's communication, which will be profound once he or she realizes that we can be trusted, that our openness and patience are really a gift of love and not a means of manipulation.

Listening to another, really listening, is the greatest gift of love that we can give.

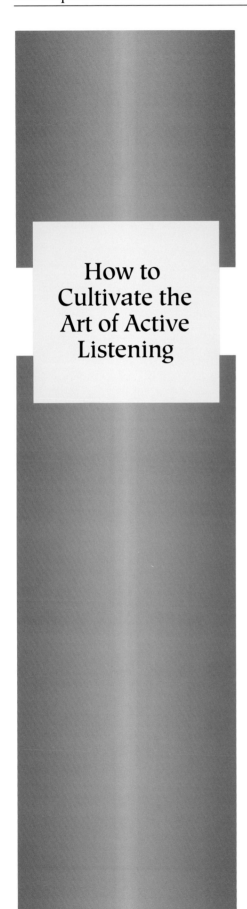

# How to Cultivate the Art of Active Listening

Listening is at the heart of all communication, yet, as we have seen, most of us listen only partially. Then, because we haven't taken time to hear the whole story, we make assumptions or jump to conclusions that are not necessarily true. We call true listening "active" because it takes energy and time. If you don't feel you have those in the moment that listening is called for, say so, and arrange to get together when you do have the necessary energy and time.

There are many benefits, both for you and the other, from listening well: you come to learn more of who the other person is; you allow the other to feel understood and accepted by you; you hear yourself reflected in the other person; you help him or her solve his or her own problems; and you create an atmosphere of love and trust that sets the stage for fulfilling ongoing communication between the two of you. You also reduce his or her anxiety and allow him or her to feel comfortable sharing with you, thus creating greater friendship and love.

Here is what you need to do to be an active listener:
1. Take time to really listen.
2. Sit in a relaxed, receptive way.
3. Establish and maintain eye contact.
4. Sit at the same eye level (physical equality).
5. Remind yourself that the person is worthy of respect and attention. (Think of all the good things you know about that person.)
6. Drop your expectations and fears about what you're going to say or do.
7. Really hear the person.
8. Be present (do not allow yourself to be distracted).
9. Be natural.
10. Be patient.
11. Try to feel the other person empathetically — what is he or she experiencing? (Empathy means "to feel with.")
12. Drop your own responses, rationalizations, justifications, and explanations, and just listen. Allow the person to express his or her feelings without your mental "but's" or verbal interjections. Hear him or her out.

## Barriers to Active Listening

What can interfere with our ability to listen actively?

Conscious and unconscious barriers can arise externally or within our minds and interfere with our ability to listen to another person. Some examples of those kinds of barriers are the following:
1. Distractions in the environment.
2. Excessive worry about our own problems or concerns.
3. Fear of criticism from the other person.
4. Unfinished business. (For example, "I'm still reacting to what you did yesterday, so I can't really hear what you're saying now.")
5. Second-guessing. (For example, "I already know what you're going to say, so I have turned off my attention.")
6. Not being with this person. (For example, "I'm not really seeing you; I'm seeing someone you remind me of, so I'm hearing his/her voice instead of yours.")

Active listening means true acceptance of the other person . . . exactly as he or she is.

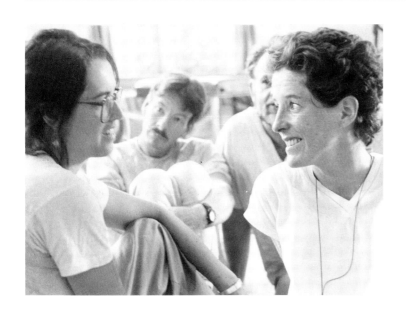

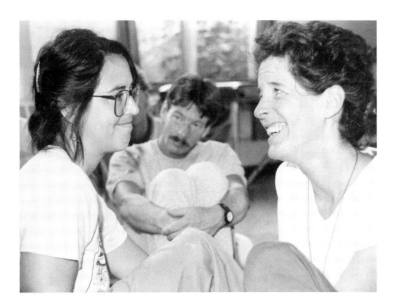

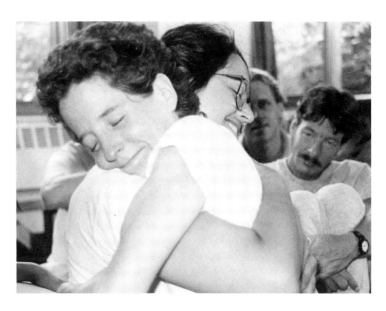

# Beyond Clear Communication

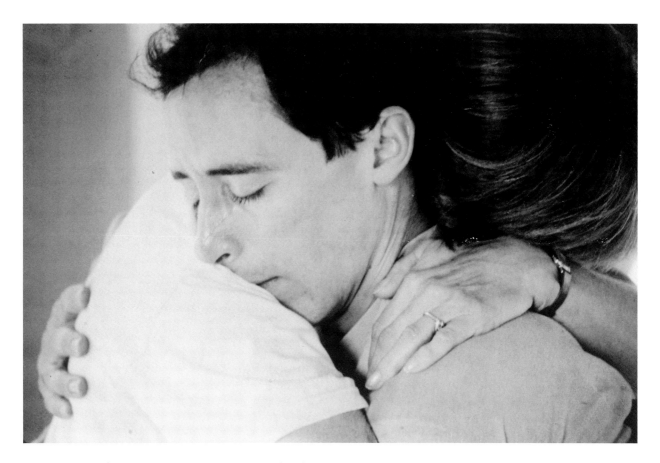

After learning to communicate clearly, our next step is to learn to communicate lovingly. Once we know what it is we feel, we must learn to find words that express our feeling in a way that is both honest and loving. It is good to recognize that we are angry; it is not so good to express that anger by shouting or speaking in a hostile way to the person who is its target, because that will make it more difficult for clear and loving communication to happen between us.

The following is a series of pointers excerpted from the teachings of Yogi Desai on how to see your communications with others as a way to love them more.

# LOVE'S COMMUNICATION
## by Yogi Amrit Desai

Failure to communicate is not verbal inability so much as lack of attunement or lack of love for the other. Love communicates better than words because the feeling is transmitted directly. No matter how good the words, without love your message will not get across. The other person will be deaf to your logic and even to the truth, until you add a little love. So instead of trying to explain, try to love.

Communicating in a clear way is a gift, not only to yourself, but to others. By helping others to understand you, you are opening them up to life. You are providing them with new ears, enabling them to hear and understand another person.

On the contrary, your inability to communicate clearly does not merely result in your not getting a message across; you are closing the others down and shutting off their experience of you and the world simply by not choosing the right words. You may well create enemies, even though your intentions are good, if you don't use the right language. So learning how to communicate well is a first step in learning how to love unconditionally.

A principle of human nature that is very deeply rooted is the craving to be appreciated. If you can fulfill that craving in someone else, then you have really communicated. Of course that fulfillment should only be offered with the highest motive — the pure selfless desire to help and to extend love to the other.

If you can be unattached in your communication and your motive is pure and selfless, you will have no difficulty being heard, because what you want from that person, if it is based on unconditional love and understanding, is the same as his own higher nature wants for him or her. Appeal to the highest instincts in the other and you will draw out the highest response.

If you speak softly, gently, and truthfully, you develop a silent strength in your language and it will have the ring of truth when you speak. If you watch your thoughts, taking care to harbor only kind, loving, and truthful thoughts, they too will have power.

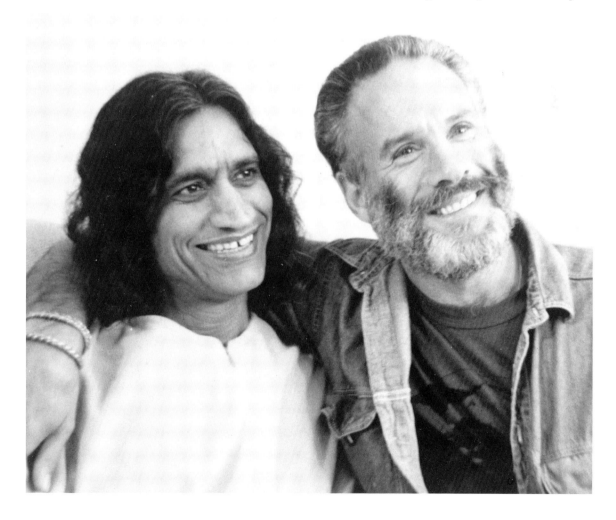

People who are in the habit of lying and being dishonest have very confused minds. They are always restless, tense, and fearful, so no one pays much attention to what they say.

It is important to be accurate and specific when you speak. To generalize and exaggerate is very harmful to your consciousness because your subconscious mind is not discriminating: it takes everything you say literally.

Always speak and think positively about other people. This gives them freedom to change. If you criticize and condemn others, you are reinforcing their weakness and giving it deeper roots. If you find it difficult to speak well of others always, it is because you don't really want to change. If you are willing to grow and to be flexible, you will allow that to others too.

Be economical in your speech. Say only what is necessary and avoid wasting energy in unnecessary emotional expressions. When you use your energy to express negative emotions, it sets up a negative reverberation within you.

When you experience negative or unpleasant emotions, the most important thing to recognize is that it is natural and normal to feel those emotions at times. So you have every right to experience what you are feeling. But you don't have the right to impose it on others. So you must take care to explain to them at that time, in a courteous way, that you are experiencing a negative emotion that is clouding your ability to communicate with them.

If you tell others that you are experiencing a negative emotion and don't want to project it onto them, they will accept it. If instead you impose your anger on them, you will simply receive anger in return. If you are able to express your negative feelings positively and objectively, you will reap positive benefits for yourself.

All negative emotions, such as anger, hatred, and jealousy, come from one source: you wanted something from that person and didn't get it. Remember that the more specifications you have about how life should be, the more occasions you will have to get angry.

Do not try to get sympathy from others for what you see as problems in your life. Sympathy will simply make you feel justified in your current position and you will not accept the responsibility for your emotions or take the opportunity to grow through the understanding of them. Accept your negative feelings without spreading them, knowing that they will not last. They are a part of life and growth, just as storms are part of the life of our environment.

After accepting your negative emotions, the next step is to work to understand them: to find out where they come from and see clearly what part your selfish interests play in them. When you begin to be objective about negative feelings, you will find them dissolving, for they are only the result of misunderstanding.

When you are afraid to try to understand your negative emotions, you lose the capacity to be objective; obviously, you don't want to face your fear. Being afraid of fear, however, doubles it. If you can face a fear fairly and squarely, once and for all, instead of avoiding or ignoring it, then it will never come back to haunt you.

Remember that just as you are growing in awareness, so is everyone else, in his or her own way. It may not look like your way. It may not even be apparent to you. But there is an inner evolutionary urge in all of us. So remember the prayer of St. Francis and, instead of wanting to be understood, try to understand the other person and say, "You're doing it your way and that's fine."

You will never get complete understanding from others, because no one can understand you the way you understand yourself. And you may never fully understand others. But it is within your power to accept others as they are and to love them.

When love exists, communication of the highest order occurs spontaneously. Communication then is really a communion flowing from heart to heart rather than from head to head. That is true communication.

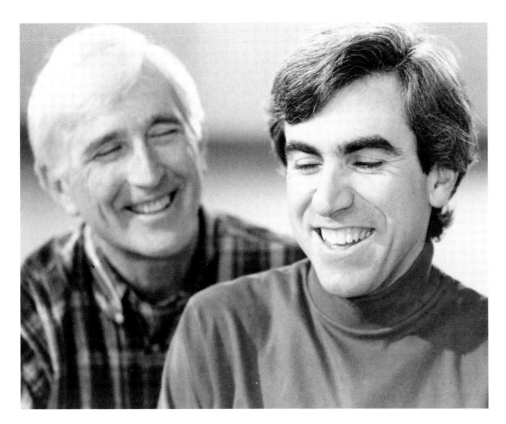

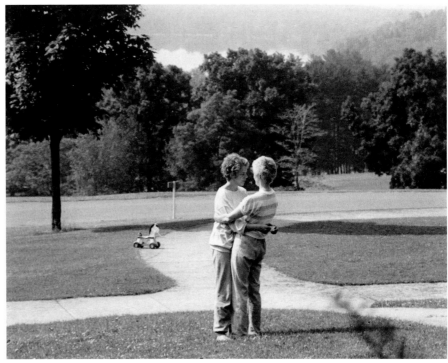

# How to Express Feelings and Give Feedback

As we have seen, expressing feelings is, for most of us, much harder than expressing opinions, facts, or theories. If you listen to people's conversations, you will notice that usually they are either describing things, events, or people (it may be books, movies, politics, or friends) or exchanging facts and opinions about those topics. Very rarely are conversations about personal feelings, because talking about feelings involves a risk.

Because we have accepted the general world-view that says our feelings are who we are, expressing those feelings means revealing our inner selves. If the other person does not like the self we think we are, we may also find it difficult to like and accept that self. It seems particularly risky if the feelings we are revealing are those commonly labeled "negative," "weak," or "unacceptable," such as anger, frustration, or hurt. And for some people it is simply not considered appropriate to discuss feelings at all.

Part of the reason that we're reluctant to express our feelings to others is that we do not feel confident of our ability to say what we feel in a way that is both honest and, at the same time, loving and kind. Experience has taught us that if we do not succeed in finding the correct words and tone of voice to give feedback about our feelings, then we may provoke anger, hostility, or hurt in the other person.

Out of fear of imagined consequences, we often remain silent even when we believe it would be useful to give feedback. As a result, we bottle up our feelings and then may harbor resentment because of them, or lose our tempers later and express the feelings in a way that provokes the very reaction we originally feared.

Giving feedback and expressing feelings can be an easy and rewarding experience if we learn a few simple guidelines and a slightly new point of view. The result of being able to give feedback lovingly and clearly is a sense of release and freedom and a new openness between us and others. It also fosters a fresh and often unforeseen liking and respect, instead of distance and fear.

Here are some guidelines for giving feedback, structured in the Three A's format.

## Awareness

1. Become aware of what you are feeling. It is very important to recognize clearly the feeling that you wish to share. Simply knowing that you feel upset or uncomfortable will not enable you to become clear about the nature of your feelings. You will need to refine your awareness until you can be more precise and say to yourself, "I feel hurt (or appreciated, unloved, loved, unconsidered, afraid, confident, angry, or whatever it is)."

2. Understand and accept the true origin of your feelings. Often we make the mistake of believing that we are experiencing a certain feeling because someone else did something and "made" us feel that way. Remember that we are the creators of our feelings and experiences. It is our interpretation of the other person's acts or words that causes us to feel the way we do, not the acts themselves.

The idea that we alone are responsible for our feelings is a hard one for many of us to get. Yet we must be able to accept it fully and wholeheartedly if we are to express our feelings and feedback objectively and lovingly. It is only our past conditioning that makes us believe that we experience hurt, anger, or pain because of someone else's actions.

Once we take back the responsibility for what we are feeling, we experience a tremendous power in our lives. We no longer feel like a victim or bystander; we no longer give others the power to decide how we experience our lives. Also, the others in our lives will be more open to us when they see that we no longer blame them for what we are feeling, and they will be more willing to assume responsibility for their own feelings.

Ask yourself about a specific situation that has brought up feelings for you:

(a)   What do I believe or imagine that the other person is telling me through his or her words and actions?

(b)   How is my feeling a result of that belief? In actual fact, the other person may not have meant what you imagined, so you may have a pleasant surprise when you check it out with him or her.

3. Once you are clear on the first two points, examine your motivation for sharing your feelings. If what you really want is some result from your sharing, your feedback will not be as well received as you would like.

Often we tell ourselves that we simply want to let others know how we are feeling, when in fact, deep down, we really want them to change their behavior so that it is more acceptable to us or to make them feel responsible, or even guilty, for the way they have "made" us feel. Either of those is a perfectly understandable and human reaction that we may not even recognize because we think it is "bad" and, therefore, believe we should not feel that way.

However, once we see and accept that motivation, we are freed to go on to the next step, which is to find a more loving and objective reason for sharing our feelings. Some positive reasons for giving feed-back to others might be any of the following:

(a)   to learn whether they meant what you imagined they meant;

(b)   to clarify a miscommunication or situation so that it will not occur again;

(c)   to reveal yourself to others fearlessly and openly, as you are, so that they know you better and are also able to be more open with you;

(d)   to provide them with objective information on their environment so that they can decide whether or not to modify their words or behavior in order to interact more harmoni-ously with others. (You will have to be open to the possibility that others may choose not to change and you must be sure you feel okay with that. It is, after all, their right.)

## Acceptance

4. Accept full responsibility for creating your feelings — through beliefs created by past experiences causing you to react in the way you do — and you will gradually be able to accept complete responsibility for your life. You will also begin to feel very free.

5. Accept the other person's response. It may be that no matter how objective and loving your feedback is, the other person will still not be open to hearing it. That is usually because he or she has his or her own internal agenda or misconceptions about what you are saying and why. Your ability to accept reaction to your feedback with equanimity is proof of your original objectivity.

If you feel frustrated, hurt, or angry at the response to your feedback, ask yourself "What is it I wanted from the exchange? How did I expect or want the person to respond?" In that way, giving feedback is a means of learning more about yourself as well as giving the other person the opportunity to learn more about you and about him- or herself.

Feedback involves taking risks: the risk of learning something about yourself that you didn't know before (and that you may not initially feel comfort-able with) and the risk of being misunderstood or not accepted. Yet those are worthwhile risks, because you also stand to gain a new love, understanding, and respect from yourself and from others for your fearlessness in showing yourself just as you are.

## Adjustment

6. You are about ready to give your feedback. Before you do, check it against the list of criteria that fol-lows, to ensure that it meets all the requirements for objective and loving communication. As you do this ongoingly, you will experience a growing confidence in your ability to express your feelings to others in a clear way.

# Loving and Objective Feedback...

## 1. Is asked for, or agreed to, willingly.

Feedback is most helpful and openly received when it has been asked for. If it has not been requested, at least ask the person whether or not he or she is willing to hear you.

**FOR EXAMPLE:**

*Imposed feedback:* "I need to share something with you right now."

*A way to seek agreement:* "I have some feelings that I think would be helpful for me to share with you. Would you be willing to listen to them? When would be a good time?"

## 2. Is well-timed.

Although feedback is most helpful right after the situation has occurred, other factors must be considered. Is the situation appropriate for the giving of feedback immediately? Is the other person ready and willing to hear it then?

**FOR EXAMPLE:**

*Ill-timed feedback:* "I have to tell you that I got really angry at you this morning when . . . oh dear! I didn't realize you had a hard time with your boss at the office today. I didn't mean to upset you."

*Well-timed feedback:* "Thanks for agreeing to this time when I can share with you. I feel more comfortable knowing you are rested and relaxed."

## 3. Owns responsibility.

As discussed above, blaming others only results in their feeling defensive and closed to you. It is more helpful to use statements that show clearly that you accept that your feelings are a result of your interpretation of the other's actions.

**FOR EXAMPLE:**

*Blaming the other:* "You make me so angry when you come home late for supper."

*Accepting responsibility:* "When you come home late for supper, I imagine that you don't care about my feelings, and as a result of imagining that I get upset."

A Tip: To help you to remain with your own responsibility, use statements beginning with "I" as much as possible, rather than with "you" or "it."

**FOR EXAMPLE:**

*Instead of* "It makes me mad . . . ," *say* "I get mad . . ."

*Instead of* "You really have to laugh when . . . ," *say* "I really have to laugh when . . ."

*Instead of* "One can't help being upset when . . . ," *say* "I become upset when . . ."

*Instead of* "We all make mistakes," *say* "I make mistakes."

*Instead of* "People do the silliest things," *say* "I do the silliest things."

Notice the different feeling you have when you make the statement in the second way, where you are really owning the feelings involved rather than making general statements about life that are intellectual rather than experiential.

## 4. Checks out the other's feelings and intentions.

Ask questions that verify where others were coming from when they spoke/acted, rather than making statements ascribing motives to them that may be totally inaccurate.

**FOR EXAMPLE:**

*Making assumptions about others' feelings:* "I wish you wouldn't be so impatient with me."

*Checking it out:* "When you spoke to me just now I imagined you were feeling impatient with me. Is that accurate, or was something else happening?"

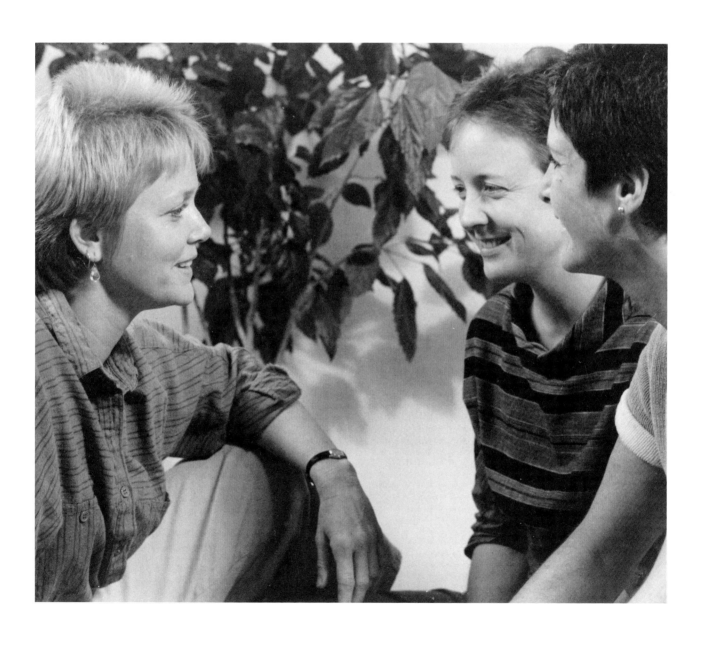

## 5. Is descriptive rather than evaluative.

Describing your own feelings without placing a value judgement on the actions or words of the other leaves him or her free to respond without defensiveness or rationalization.

### FOR EXAMPLE:

*Evaluative:* "It is so inconsiderate of you to always keep me waiting when we are going somewhere."

*Descriptive:* "It seems to me that you are often late when we are going somewhere, and I must admit that I don't like to wait for people. Can we work this out together?"

## 6. Is specific rather than general.

This helps the other person not to feel always in the wrong and shows that it is not the person that you are unhappy with, but simply an aspect of behavior.

### FOR EXAMPLE:

*General:* "You always try to dominate the situation."

*Specific:* "Just now when you said that, I imagined that you did not want to listen to what I had to say, and I felt unhappy."

## 7. Takes into account the receiver's needs also.

The receiver of your feedback will be more open to your feelings if you show that you are open to his or her needs too.

### FOR EXAMPLE:

*Takes into account the speaker's needs only:* "I don't like it when you wake me up early in the morning."

*Takes the receiver's needs into account also:* "I don't like it when you wake me up early, yet I do understand your need to get up at that time. Can we work out a compromise?"

## 8. Is checked afterward.

There are two good reasons for checking back to see how your communication was received. First, you ensure that the other person has really understood what you wanted him or her to understand, and second, you find out how he or she is feeling about what you have shared. In other words, you get feedback on your feedback!

### FOR EXAMPLE:

*Unverified communication:* "Well, that's all I wanted to say; thanks for listening."

*Verified:* "Please tell me what you heard me say, so that I can be sure I communicated clearly. And how do you feel about what we have just shared?"

## 9. Is directed toward behavior the receiver can do something about if he or she chooses to.

This avoids generating a feeling of frustration or even despair in the receiver.

### FOR EXAMPLE:

*Directed at something unchangeable/irrational:* "The way you talk to me makes me unhappy because it reminds me of my mother. She always talked like that."

*Directed at changeable behavior:* "When you spoke to me just now, you seemed rather abrupt and impatient and I felt threatened. I realize it is just an old habit pattern being activated: it reminded me of the way my mother sometimes spoke. As a child I felt anxious at those times, because I thought she didn't love me. I wanted to tell you that background so that you can understand my reaction better. Would you be willing to speak less abruptly to me to help me take in what you're saying?"

The examples above will give you a feel for ways that you can take more responsibility for your feelings so that others are comfortable when you share with them. As you master your communication, you will find that others begin to welcome your feedback, because they trust your objectivity and enjoy getting to know you better. Often it comes as a great relief to both sides to know how the other is feeling; usually it is not nearly so dark a picture as we imagine! Also, you will come to feel really good about yourself as your capacity to be more open with others increases.

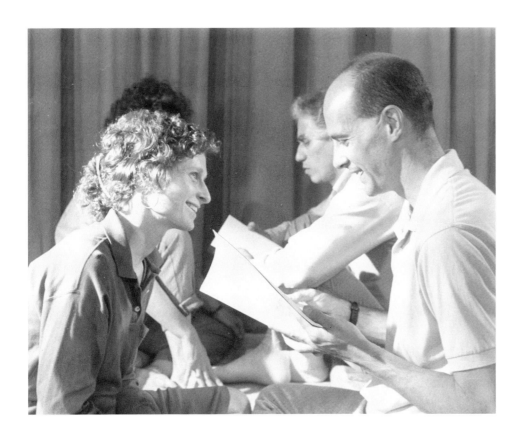

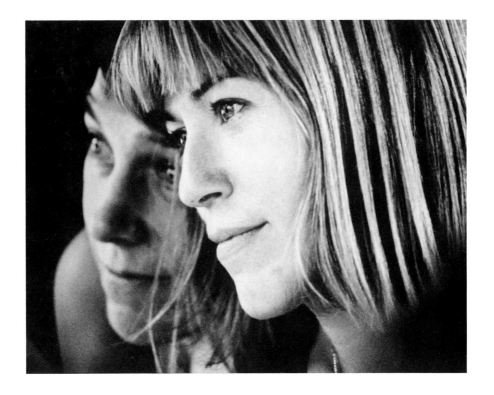

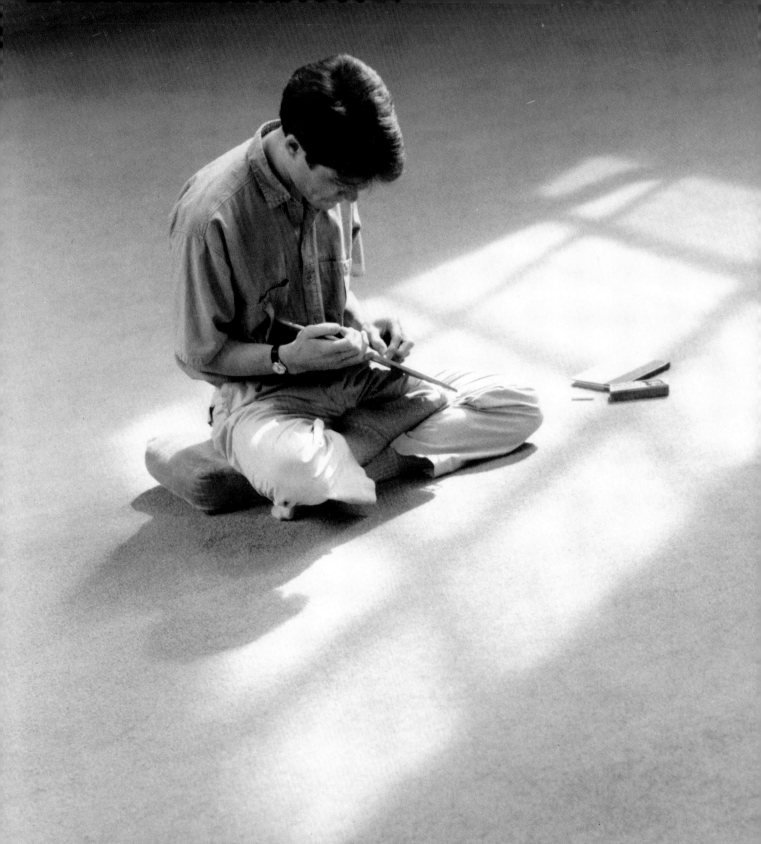

# The Seventh Pathway

practicing meditation and spiritual attunement

# What Is Spiritual Attunement?

You may not use those words to describe it, but there is no doubt that you have experienced many moments of spiritual attunement in your life. Such moments come in varying ways, depending on your temperament, your lifestyle, and your beliefs.

Perhaps there was a moment when you felt completely at peace with the world, when everything seemed to be unfolding as it should and your every need seemed to be met, your every desire stilled or fulfilled. Or you may have experienced it in a timeless moment of ecstasy and joy at the beauty of nature, as you walked in the mountains or by the ocean at sunset.

Perhaps one of your moments of attunement has been a calm sensation of warmth, fulfillment, and gratitude, as you sat with ones you love. Maybe it came to you as a feeling of profound satisfaction and absorption as you completed a work of art or even a simple craft, and gloried in your creative energies. Or it may have come to you in a place of worship or in private prayer.

There are as many ways to experience spiritual attunement as there are people in the world and each way is satisfying — for that moment. The problem is that experiences like those described above are of limited duration. After them we are plunged once again into the work-a-day world with all its intense stimulations and perceived difficulties.

That need not be the case, however. Spiritual attunement, like other states, can be cultivated. We can learn to make that deeply satisfying and joyful feeling part of our everyday life. In fact, the experience of peace, joy, and satisfaction is our birthright as human beings, not a special blessing only conferred on us occasionally.

The basic ingredient of spiritual attunement seems to be a feeling of completeness, of oneness or unity. Or, if oneness is not a conscious ingredient, at least there is the absence of conflict or dis-ease: the experiences of the body, the thoughts of the mind, and the aspirations of the spirit are all in harmony.

The question is how can we bring that harmony into our lives more often? What do we need to do?

## Your Instrument of Attunement: Your Body, Mind, and Spirit

Imagine for a moment that you are a violinist, about to take your seat with an orchestra to play a symphony. How do you prepare yourself? First you must make certain that all the strings of your instrument are at the correct tension or the sounds they make will be nothing more than dull twanging. So each separate string must be tuned to its appropriate pitch.

Then the strings have to be tuned to each other. However beautiful each string sounds when played alone, if it is not tuned to the other three, the result will still not be music and harmony, but discord and harshness.

When that is accomplished and you take your seat with the orchestra, you still need to tune your instrument to the instruments of those with whom you are about to play or, again, the result will not be harmony. The group attunement is achieved by having each instrument tune to one standard, universal pitch.

Now see the violin as a symbol for a human being. The human instrument has three strings: body, mind, and spirit. Each string needs to be perfectly tuned within itself first: The body must be perfectly healthy and the mind clear and objective; the spirit must be recognized as pure and free.

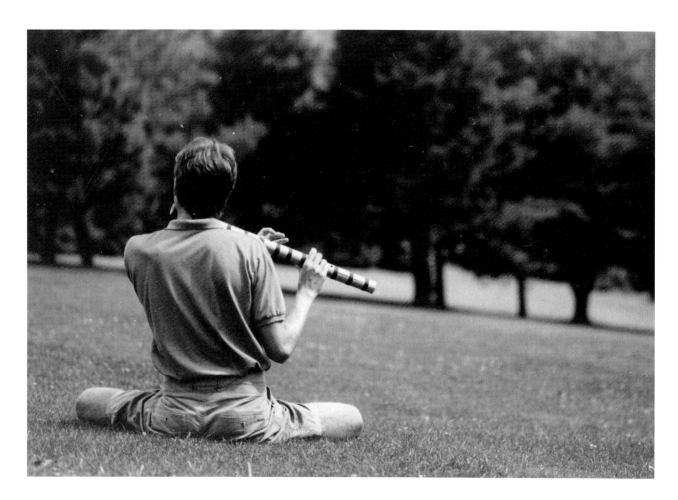

Then the three strings must be tuned to each other. In both our example of the violin and in the human, one string serves as the base or ground against which the others are tuned. In the human being that ground is the spirit — our indwelling prana in its most subtle manifestation.

Once we bring our body and mind into attunement with our prana, through the many methods suggested in this book, we will find that we are unerringly attuned to all that surrounds us, for we are in harmony with the pitch of nature itself, the vibration of the universe. Individual prana always resonates in harmony with universal prana.

The key to all health, peace, and happiness, then, is learning how to attune our body and mind to our prana, at every moment of the day. There are two levels on which we can work to bring about the alignment of body and mind with the knowingness of spirit: The first is the practice of specific techniques and the second is a heightening of our daily awareness of the voice of prana.

The material that follows includes an explanation of the use of meditation as a tool for spiritual awareness and an article by Yogi Desai about a unique way to be aware of our thoughts and movements in daily life, so that life becomes an expression of spirit.

# Self-Discovery Experience

# 14

## Attuning to your higher self

## Awareness

1. Take an inner inventory. Close your eyes for a moment and get in touch with times, places, and circumstances in which you felt truly in tune with your inner Self. Then list them freely, allowing your mind to acknowledge even the briefest and most subtle moments of being close to the being you really are.

2. Arrange your list in order of frequency of occurrence. Which five attunement experiences are the most frequent?

3. Go back to your original list and now arrange it in order of the potency of the experience. Which five attunement experience are the most powerful?

4. Are the five most frequent the same or different from the five most powerful?

## Acceptance

5. Consider how often you find or put yourself in your five most powerful attunement experiences.

6. Examine one that you would like to experience more often. Explore any tendencies in yourself, your habits, or your attitudes that affect how often you practice that form of attunement.

7. Close your eyes once again and attune to your inner wisdom now, allowing yourself to receive compassionate guidance. Ask your higher self: "How should I go about attuning myself more to your needs? Show me where I am neglecting you and how I can express you more clearly."

## Adjustment

8. Reflect on the guidance. Ask for specific, practical ways to implement it and write them down.

9. Consider how friends or loved ones might be able to assist you in creating more times and circumstances for your inner attunement. Sincerely share your needs and aspirations with them, giving them the opportunity to ask questions or make suggestions. With flexibility and a common purpose, you are sure to achieve a harmonious integration of their needs and yours.

# MEDITATION AND THE SEARCH FOR PEACE OF MIND

### by Yogi Amrit Desai

## Getting "Enough"

We are all searching, in our different ways, for lasting peace of mind. Few people are fortunate enough to find it. Many things seem to block the way to inner peace. The first is the belief that peace of mind depends on external, material security. People say "I want to live in peace and enjoy life, but I must have security for that. I must have enough security to provide adequately for myself and my family."

What do the words *enough* and *adequate* really mean? How much is enough? How will you know when you have enough external security? Is it when it gives you complete peace of mind? If so, you will never get enough. It will never give you the peace of mind you seek, because external, material security and success alone are not capable of providing you with true, lasting peace of mind.

Look around you. There are so many people who still do not have peace of mind even after achieving what they and others think of as great success and material security. For years, those people have looked forward to retiring with enough time and resources to experience freedom from worry and really enjoy life.

But when the time comes for retirement and they, indeed, have the luxury of material resources and time to enjoy life to the fullest, what happens? The cherished dream turns into a nightmare for many. Their freedom becomes the worst form of punishment: They are totally unable to enjoy it because they do not possess the key to the enjoyment of leisure time — peace of mind.

## Security or Serenity?

Such people are so restless that they are completely unable to enjoy a relaxed life. They have developed an unbreakable habit of needing activity, of needing problems to solve and things to do all day long. They became so preoccupied with their search for enough success and security that, without realizing it, they sacrificed both their health and their peace of mind.

Now that they have enough material security, they have neither the physical health nor the mental peace to enjoy it. They have traded serenity for security. It is a poor exchange.

So the search for peace of mind through the acquisition of material security is an illusion. Such a life is like that of a mouse running on a treadmill. There is no freedom. The only choice you have is to run faster or slower. The faster you run, the more you are blind to what is happening around and within you. And there is no point of arrival — ever.

## Peace of Mind, Now

That does not mean you should give up all concern for material security for yourself and your family. Not at all. Simply recognize that external security will never bring you the lasting peace of mind that you seek.

Ask yourself "What is the true meaning of security to me? Is it simply external success and material prosperity? Or does it also concern my state of mind? My physical health? My emotional well-being? Is it for the future, or is it for now as well?" When you have the answers to those questions, ask one more: "Do I need to change my life, or my attitude, to provide myself with the peace of mind I seek — right now?"

Peace of mind, like restlessness and dissatisfaction, is a habit. It is either nurtured or destroyed by how you live each moment of each day of your life. It comes from within you, not from external objects or events. Because it is an attitude, it can be cultivated. Because it is a habit, it can be acquired through constant repetition and practice.

Meditation is one of the most powerful tools available to human beings in their search for lasting peace of mind. Meditation helps on two levels. First, it helps you to go within yourself and find, in the peaceful depths of your being, answers to all your questions and searching. Second, it brings balance and clarity to your mind and strength to your will, qualities that enable you to transform your old habits of restlessness and tension into new patterns of health-giving peace and self-fulfillment.

## The Searching Mind

Meditation works in the following way. The mind is, by its very nature, restless and searching. First, it divides all experiences into two categories: pleasurable and unpleasurable, or painful. It then seeks out pleasure and satisfaction, which it hopes to find from external objects, events, and people and internal memories of objects, events, and people. At the same time, it tries to avoid painful experiences and memories.

The stronger its likes and dislikes, the more restless and overactive the mind is. Strong likes and dislikes generate strong emotions, and the stronger the emotions, the greater the energy they consume. Strong emotions are blinding: they prevent the mind from seeing truth objectively and making the best decisions.

A mind that is swayed by strong likes and dislikes is unable to find solutions to even the easiest of problems; its confusion complicates the simplest situations.

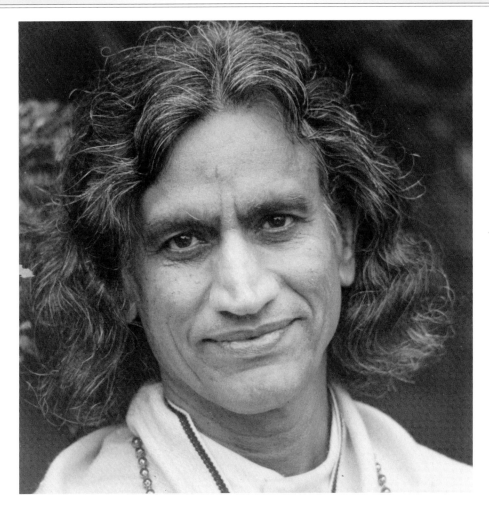

We have all experienced that. Even the wisest people are capable of acting foolishly when their minds are swayed by conflicting emotions, desires, or fears. They have no access to their store of wisdom when their minds are restless and unsettled.

Meditation, then, calms and focuses the restless mind. A steady, calm mind opens the door to all wisdom and knowledge, because prana can flow freely through it, just as prana flows more freely through a relaxed body. Prana, remember, is the universal life force, the universal mind, the source of all wisdom and knowledge. A restless mind is a veil between us and that universal source of knowledge.

As soon as the mind is calmed and emptied of conflicting thoughts and desires, true wisdom and knowledge begin to flow into the space created. This emptying is the source of all creativity, intuition, and wisdom. As your mind becomes calm and still and you enter into the depths of your being, you will contact that universal intelligence in your heart as an experience of peace and love.

## Emptying the Mind to Receive Wisdom

So meditation is the process of emptying the mind so that it can receive universal wisdom, peace, and love, which paradoxically is already there, deep within you, just waiting to be contacted.

In meditation you begin to dissolve your restlessness, your intense likes and dislikes, and your attachments and fears. You no longer see life in terms of opposites to be sought or avoided. Ultimately, when it is mastered, meditation becomes a spontaneously experienced state of thought-free stillness and ecstasy. In order to reach that level, specific techniques must be practiced to tame the restless mind that has had a lifetime of unfettered activity. All meditation techniques have one common goal: to help meditators achieve the stillness of mind that will allow them to make deep contact with their inner source of wisdom, peace, and fulfillment.

Beginning meditation techniques are more properly called concentration techniques. Concentration techniques focus the thoughts that are normally scattered into many different directions, diffusing the energy of the mind and causing tension and restlessness. Concentration focuses the scattered energy and focused energy leads to the experience of inner peace and calm.

A form of concentration-meditation is described in the following way by the great yogi, Patanjali, in about the 4th century B.C.: "Meditation occurs when all thoughts begin to flow in an unbroken chain toward one subject, without interruption from thoughts of unrelated subjects."

Concentration can be on any subject, mundane or spiritual. Whatever the subject, the mind is trained to focus its energies on a single subject. Meditation, on the other hand, focuses on subjects that are spiritually inspiring. Its purpose is to awaken the meditator to higher states of awareness and spiritual consciousness.

## Kripalu Yoga Meditation in Motion

There are many different types and techniques of meditation, each suitable to a certain temperament and level of spiritual development. Classical seated meditation, known as Raja Yoga, is usually practiced after a certain level of physical skill in Hatha Yoga postures has been attained.

Kripalu Yoga is different from either of those practices, yet combines the benefits of both. It also eliminates the drawbacks they sometimes hold for Westerners. It has been my privilege to originate and develop Kripalu Yoga as a technique especially suited to the Western temperament, which is highly active, both physically and mentally.

When many Westerners practice seated Raja Yoga meditation, their bodies become restless after a while and that is a distraction from meditation. On the other hand, when they are practicing Hatha Yoga, they are often not taught to concentrate their minds sufficiently on the postures, with the result that their thoughts roam restlessly and they do not gain full benefit from the exercises. In both cases peace of mind and a deeply meditative state are elusive.

In Kripalu Yoga, the body movements themselves are the focus of concentration. Through specific ways of moving and breathing (see the section on Kripalu Yoga in the Second Pathway: Getting to Know and Love Your Body) a powerful magnetic field is created that keeps the mind totally concentrated on the movements being performed and results in a deeply meditative state being attained almost effortlessly. Kripalu Yoga, then, leads you in five stages from the level of simple concentration to the transcendent stage where both meditation and movement are spontaneous. At that level you experience an intense awareness of the divine nature of prana and a deep sense of inner peace, contentment, and fulfillment.

## The Benefits of Meditation

The regular practice of meditation will bring profound and far-reaching benefits to your life, no matter what your age or background. First you will begin to experience a level of physical relaxation and inner peace that you have not previously known, a peace that continues long after the period of actual meditation.

Your mind will become clearer, more focused, and more powerful, enabling you to make decisions and take action with greater ease. Your creativity and intuitive powers will be awakened. You will find yourself gaining the ability to remain calm even in the midst of stressful and conflicting situations.

As a result of increased calmness, you will experience a greater ability to accept things as they are, including other people and yourself. So your interpersonal relationships will become more successful and harmonious.

All the above benefits will come from the regular practice of short periods of meditation. For those interested in holistic health, Kripalu Yoga's Meditation in Motion is the ideal form of meditation because it works with the whole person: body, mind and spirit. It is a holistic meditation.

# Three Simple Meditation Techniques

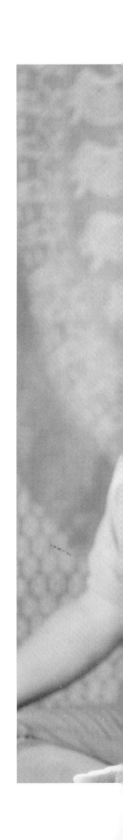

Three meditation techniques are described here. The first, and simplest, will give you a feel for the basic elements of meditation. You can then apply those basics as you experiment with the other two.

Remember, however, that the key to progress in meditation is to pick one technique and practice it regularly, rather than skipping from technique to technique. At one of his seminars on Yoga, Consciousness, and Love, Yogi Desai was asked by a seminar participant, "What is the best technique for meditation?" Without a moment's hesitation he replied, "The one you're practicing!"

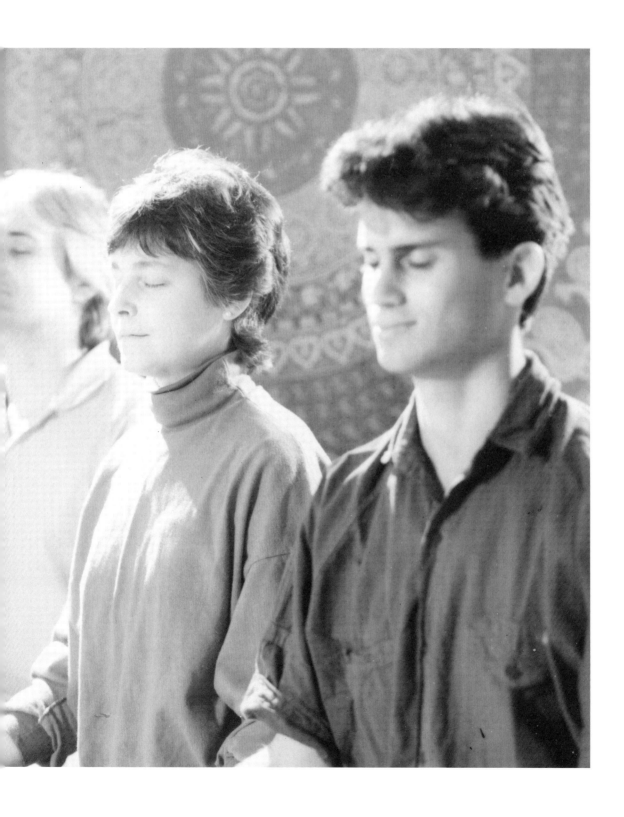

## Preparing for Meditation

In each of the techniques described, the prerequisites are the same.

1. Choose a quiet, secluded place where you will not be interrupted or disturbed.

2. Choose a time when you can sit for meditation each day, so that it becomes a positive habit. You will find as you become constant in your practice that your mind and body will learn to become quieter and more introspective at that time every day.

3. Dim the lights and, if you like, light candles and/or incense to create a conducive environment.

4. Shower or bathe before meditating, or at least wash your face, hands, and feet to increase your receptivity.

5. Wear clean clothes (some meditators choose white clothing) to help create a vibration of specialness and of calm and peace, a feeling of being lifted for awhile out of the usual pace of external life activity.

6. Have near you when you meditate one or more inspiring pictures of people or deities whom you love and respect, those who symbolize for you the state of inner peace and tranquility that you want to contact.

7. Relax as much as you can before you begin, using the techniques suggested in this book. Then sit in a comfortable position, spine erect, chin parallel to the floor and tucked in slightly. Sitting cross-legged on the floor is best, or kneeling on a meditation bench.

   It is more important to be comfortable than to be correct, however, so if you need a chair, use one. If you use a chair, sit with both feet on the floor and your arms by your sides.

   Place your hands either palms up on your thighs or lightly clasped in your lap. Make certain that your shoulders are dropped back and relaxed and that your neck is loose (rotate it if necessary, to relax it). Close your eyes and begin to take long, slow, deep yogic breaths (see page 76 for instruction on Yogic Deep Breathing).

## Meditation on the Sound of Om

In this meditation, we practice focusing the mind on the sound of *Om*, which has been considered for centuries to be particularly relaxing and centering.

1. Prepare as above and sit quietly for a few minutes. Drop all expression from your face and consciously relax the various parts of your body, especially the face, shoulders, abdomen, and hands.

2. Continue taking slow, deep breaths for two to five minutes, practicing the focusing of your total concentration on your breathing. Then gradually allow your breath to return to normal and feel yourself becoming very still within. Remain with the sensations in your body, rather than with any thoughts that may flow through your mind.

3. Mentally repeat *Om* very slowly. Feel the vibrations of the thought/sound. Listen with your whole being. After several silent, mental repetitions of the sound, very softly begin to chant the sound aloud by taking a full, deep breath in and sounding *Om* on the exhalation, making each repetition as long as is comfortably possible.

   As you continue to chant, experience the effects. Feel the peace that is created by the vibration. Imagine that the sound is flowing from deep within your abdomen and that you are opening up to let it flow out. Feel all worry, fear, and tension dissolve.

4. Remain still for a period of time, enjoying the feeling of quiet and peace within and around you. When you are ready, gradually open your eyes.

Practice this technique until you begin to feel that you are gaining some control and concentration, then move, if you wish, to a more complex technique.

## Meditation on the Internal Sound of *So'ham*

*So'ham* (pronounced "so-hahm") is an easy but powerful meditation technique that is also based on awareness of the breath. It is one of the most scientific approaches for learning the deep concentration and inner stillness necessary to experience meditation.

Take time to prepare yourself as suggested above and consciously relax the various parts of your body. Allow your consciousness of external surroundings to fade as much as possible. Then practice a few minutes of Yogic Deep Breathing, focusing your attention on the breath.

1. After approximately two to five minutes, allow the breath gradually to return to normal, keeping your concentration on it. Watch your normal flow of breath with unattached, objective awareness. Remain relaxed, not trying to control your breathing in any way. Without expectations, just watch the breath flow in and out. You will notice that the breath automatically begins to become slower and more shallow.

2. After a slow, gentle breathing rhythm is established, begin to hear, within, the sound of *so'ham* ("I am That"). Do not actually make the sound,

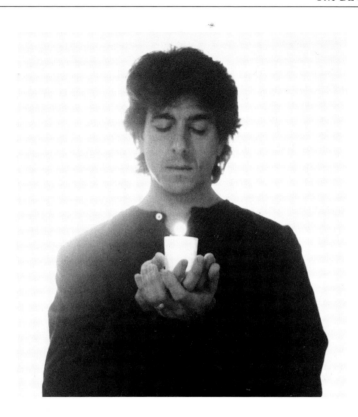

but imagine that it is the sound of the breath; "soooo" on the inhalation and "haammmm" on the exhalation. Let the breathing and the sound absorb your mind as completely as possible.

3. After a few weeks, add concentration on the point between the eyebrows (known as the "third eye"). Begin by practicing *so'ham* for about ten minutes and gradually make your sessions longer. Each time the mind wanders away from the technique, gently lead it back until the periods of mental stillness increase.

## Meditation Using Visual Concentration (*Tratak*)

*Tratak* (gazing at an object without blinking) is commonly used as a meditation technique, although it is usually classified as a yogic *kriya* (purification technique) because it strengthens and improves the eyesight and stimulates the brain cells and cranial nerves. It also, however, brings about the same benefits as other meditation techniques, partly because it develops concentration by exercising steadiness of gaze.

The following is a commonly used form of *tratak*, candle gazing. It is especially useful for beginners.

1. Use a room that is quiet and dark, with little or no air currents.
2. Place a lighted candle at eye level, making sure that it is steady and can burn safely.
3. Sit with your back straight either in a chair or cross-legged on the floor so that the position is comfortable enough to hold with a minimum of movement. Consciously relax the body and mind by using the relaxation techniques discussed above, including a few minutes of deep breathing.
4. Begin to gaze steadily into the center of the flame. As your eyes begin to water or tire, close and relax them, visualizing the flame in the space between your eyebrows. You will actually see an image left by the flame. Concentrate on that image, without mental comment, until if fades completely. Then reopen your eyes and again gaze into the flame.
5. Repeat this alternate opening and closing of the eyes, concentrating completely on each phase and dropping all other thoughts from the mind. With practice, you will find that the mind will remain still for a longer period, even after the image has faded.

When your meditation time is over, keep your eyes closed for a few minutes and relax. A good technique for relaxing the eye muscles is to rub the palms together briskly until they feel hot, then lay them across your closed eyes until they cool again. The warmth from the palms will penetrate and relax the muscles of the eyes.

Begin by limiting your meditation time to five minutes, increasing it gradually as you become more adept at the technique.

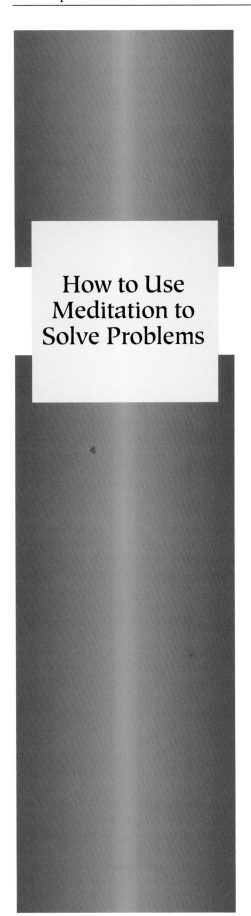

## How to Use Meditation to Solve Problems

Meditation is a profoundly effective way to solve all kinds of problems; indeed it is the most profound way for those who learn how to use it. As we progress on the path of self-development we begin to understand more and more clearly, from our own experience, the yogic truth that the solution to all problems lies within us.

It may not be easy to believe at first, but continued practice of self-awareness and self-discovery techniques, such as the ones in this book, reveals that the source of all our imagined problems does lie within our own minds as our attitudes toward the world and our habitual thinking patterns and motivations. And that is a very exciting realization, because it means that we have the power to resolve our problems and change our world.

### Tapping the Unconscious for Solutions

The solutions to what we call our problems are usually not at the level of the conscious mind, however. Like the paintings or poems of creative geniuses, creative solutions to life's problems tend to surface from deep within the unconscious without our conscious bidding. But even if we have no control over them, we are able to create circumstances that are favorable to their emergence.

Deep physical and mental relaxation and a calm mind induce the state in which solutions to problems occur to us. That is why meditation is such a powerful tool. The following method for internal problem-solving is based on the teachings of Yogi Desai. It is particularly useful when you experience a difficult interaction with another person.

In such a case, it is better not to go to the person immediately to talk about the situation, but to wait until the intense emotions have subsided. Projecting anger or negative emotions onto another is a great violence both to you and to the other. It is best to use some form of inner processing by yourself first, to become clear about the attitudes or beliefs in you that precipitated the miscommunication.

The following introspection will help you explore the situation objectively, without blaming either the other person or yourself. It will enable you simply to see the elements of the interaction as they occurred and to take responsibility (without guilt) for your part.

## Step-by-Step Instructions

1.  First, write down your feelings about the situation objectively and clearly to help you when you meditate. Ask yourself specific questions. The more clear and specific your questions, the more readily you'll come upon a solution. Look honestly at your feelings of pain, anger, or fear, or whatever the interaction brought up.

    Know that wherever there is pain, that is where your greatest attachment lies. So ask yourself now what your attachment is, what your desires in that particular situation are. You may use the same process during the meditation itself.

2.  Relax by sitting comfortably and quietly with your eyes closed. Further relax yourself by taking slow deep breaths for a few minutes.

3.  Begin to visualize, feel, or hear the voice of your Inner Teacher or Guide. Everyone has such an Inner Teacher. He or she may be the image of an external person who provides you guidance or it may be someone you've never met (perhaps someone who is not even alive now) who nevertheless inspires you in moments of need or whose teachings you follow. It may be a voice, a feeling inside, or a recognition of words of truth as they arise.

    Whatever it is, begin to feel a contact with that person or source of truth. If you visualize in images, imagine yourself seated in conversation with him or her. If you are someone who does not see images (and there are many who don't), simply become aware of any new sensations in your body and what they mean to you; in other words, use your feeling sense to make the inner contact.

4.  Begin to ask your Inner Guide, "Teach me the lesson that is hidden in this situation. What can I learn?" Share with your Inner Teacher, your Higher Self, the difficulty that you perceive in the interaction. Share objectively and clearly and feel the openness and acceptance of your Guide. At once you will feel clearer.

5.  Hold in your conscious mind the thought/image/ feeling of whatever it is you want to change. As you breathe in, image the breath and the thought rising to the spot between the eyebrows and dissolving. Do it over and over with each breath. This technique is especially effective during yogic breathing exercises.

6.  Repeat this affirmation: "I am born divine; I have no problems. All that I am perceiving in this situation is superficially imposed, artificially accepted because I have mistakenly believed in it. Now I am dropping and dissolving what I have called a problem. I no longer believe in it."

You may wish to create another specific affirmation for yourself, to help you drop and dissolve a particular problem. See the next exercise for instructions on doing that.

7.  Remain seated in meditation until you feel calmer and clearer about the situation you are processing. If one meditation does not enable you to feel completely clear and settled, you may repeat the process as many times as you need to become calm, clear, and accepting of it. Affirmations regarding the situation are also very powerful when repeated consistently over a period of time.

## Special Note

Sometimes when you process your feelings about a situation using the above technique, you may feel some strong emotions coming up. At that time, if you find it difficult to channel the energy inward, you may want to find a place where you can safely express the feelings without directing them at someone else.

You may work out feelings by beating a pillow or screaming into it, accepting that as a natural intermediate process until you can handle the feelings internally. Caution: choose a place where you will not disturb others and where they understand and accept what you are doing. A car with rolled-up windows is pretty soundproof, or you can gain surprising relief from a silent scream (going through the physical motions without making any actual sound).

Another alternative to change your energy and clear your head is to take a cold shower. You may scream again after, but do let your family or roommates know what you're doing!

## Problem Solving Using Kripalu Yoga Meditation in Motion

The location in your body where you experience physical pain when doing yoga postures corresponds to a related psychological block. That is because emotional and psychological resistances cause physical tension in the muscles of related parts of the body, such as the neck and shoulders, which in turn creates a barrier to the flow of energy. What we experience as pain is felt when the cramped muscles are stretched as the energy tries to push its way through.

So when you experience strong sensation arising, which you are tempted to call pain, first concentrate on relaxing the specific muscles involved. Then breathe into the area with a calm mind and see if any image or feeling of a related emotional or psychological issue arises. As you hold the posture, again consciously send relaxation to that area and visualize your emotional or psychological block dissolving as the muscles relax.

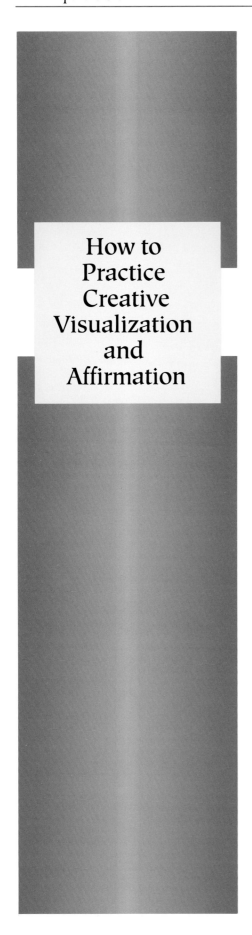

# How to Practice Creative Visualization and Affirmation

We are realizing more and more these days how easily influenced our subconscious mind is. Yet we seldom use its suggestibility in a positive, creative way to change our lives. Instead, we constantly influence the way we feel by negative reinforcements and thoughts ("I can't …" "I've never been able to …" "I'm not the kind of person who …" "I wish I could …" "If only I …")

Our subconscious minds are like children who listen to our thoughts and go about carrying them out. Simple examples show us how true that is. Let's say you're carrying a stack of dishes and start to think: "Oh dear, what if I should drop one?" The next thing you know, you do! Or you're skiing and see a rock or tree in the way and think: "I hope I don't hit that tree." No sooner has the thought entered your mind than you seem to head straight toward that very tree!

## Harnessing Our Thought Energy

This "influence-ability" of the subconscious can be a tremendous blessing if we know how to use it. The Kripalu Approach uses a technique called "Creative Visualization and Affirmation," which harnesses the power of thought energy for growth and change.

By visualizing, in your mind's eye, a situation as you would like it to unfold or yourself as you would like to be, you are creating a new formative influence on yourself to replace the old one.

The influence you generate will be as powerful as the energy of belief you put into it. If you believe it won't work, it won't, because you will not be putting enough energy into the visualization or affirmation for it to impress itself on your subconscious. Remember that thoughts are energy and energy created this universe!

It is also important to understand that you are affirming something that is already a reality. In that way affirmation is different from hypnotic suggestion. What you are affirming is true now. Your true Self (as distinct from your physical, material self of this three-dimensional plane) is perfect and complete right now: at the deepest level of your being you already are fearless, balanced, loving, and contented.

Layers of blocks may have come between the Self and your personality complex, so that the blueprint the Self provides may not have been fully executed yet in the body and mind of material form, but know that in your affirmation (for example: "I am fearless") you are speaking the absolute truth.

You are the voice of the spiritual Self speaking to your material self, your body-mind. When you accept and believe that, you will begin to make affirmations and visualizations really work for you and effect great changes in your life.

Moshe Feldenkrais, originator of the Feldenkrais Technique for body integration, has demonstrated that when people rehearse a physical action in their minds they perform it as well as, or even better than, when they have physically practiced the same action.

## The Technique of Creative Visualization and Affirmation

1. Select an area in which you would like to make changes, such as
   (a) being more relaxed;
   (b) remaining calmer when dealing with difficulties;
   (c) being more accepting of yourself and/or others;
   (d) worrying less; or
   (e) leading a healthier life.
2. Deeply relax your body and mind, using the techniques outlined earlier in this chapter.
3. Begin to see yourself in your mind's eye, as if you were looking at someone else. Picture yourself as you will be when you have changed in the way you want to. See yourself very vividly and in detail.

   Watch yourself going through a specific situation with the actions you will perform and the thoughts and feelings you will have, when you are that changed person. Hear the statements you are making at that time. See and feel other people's response to the changed you. Feel it with great intensity. Enjoy the experience deeply, feeling your joy and peace in the situation as if it were happening now.
4. Choose an affirmation that expresses the area in which you would like to change and repeat it several times, aloud if possible (if not, then mentally). Make the affirmation very simple, short, and specific. For example: "I am a capable and lovable person and I like myself" or "It is okay to make mistakes; I accept myself when I make a mistake."
5. Work on one simple and specific area until you feel you have made progress before trying another.
6. Always be very positive when you practice affirmations, selecting your words carefully. Avoid thinking of or visualizing problems or difficulties: you will only reinforce them. Stay with the positive.
7. Avoid the trap of feeling justified in your experience of the problem situation you are trying to change. The point is not to change the situation or the other people. Even if you could do so this time (and even if you are "right"), the same problem will come up again for you if it is your attitude toward the situation that is disturbing your inner peace.

If you are driving up to an intersection and have a green traffic light, but someone who has a red light is obviously not going to stop, you'd be crazy to go ahead even though you have the right of way! So seek to do what will give you peace of mind, no matter what happens. Watch how changing your attitudes changes the way you experience the world.

8. Believe that the technique of affirmation can work for you. That is very important. It is sometimes difficult for the rational mind to accept the efficacy of affirmation and visualization, yet science and psychology now have many research findings that support these techniques as effective methods to change attitudes and behavior patterns.

Most of us have accepted the fact that our unconscious minds can be "programmed" to respond in certain ways with certain behavior. Hypnotism rests on that fact. We are just beginning to realize, though, that who and what we think we are is a result of the programming we have accepted all our lives from the underlying beliefs and attitudes of our families and cultures.

## Reversing Our Programming

We have the power to undo that unconscious programming where it has had negative results. To do so, we must consciously affirm a statement of truth to replace each erroneous belief or attitude and repeat that statement enough times that it overrides the deeply imprinted negative statements we have been unconsciously "affirming" throughout our lives.

Note that it is not about replacing a negative thought with a positive one: What is vital is to affirm the truth of our beings. Because repetition of the statement is important, it is often helpful not only to think or state the affirmation, but to write it down a number of times, since that involves several of the senses at once.

It is also helpful to observe any negative responses or resistances that arise in your mind as you write the affirmations and to write them down too. Your resistances often provide seeds for further affirmations that reach an even deeper level of truth for you.

# Spiritual Attunement in Daily Life

Meditation is an essential part of a holistically healthy lifestyle because it helps us to be more attuned to our prana, which is the inner spiritual Self. The next step is extending the all-too-brief experience of meditation and its attunement to prana into our daily lives, so that we become more relaxed, balanced, flowing, and centered in whatever we do.

We are already doing that to some extent: Whenever we are totally immersed in something we love doing, such as dancing, singing, painting, or gardening, we are experiencing a form of meditation or spiritual attunement because our bodies, minds, and prana are all united and harmonized in the activity.

Those experiences, however, are few and far between for most of us. Normally we are doing one thing with our bodies while our minds are off in a totally different direction and our prana is forgotten entirely. We are not conscious of who we are, of the reality and supremacy of the inner Self. Most of us must admit that by and large we go through the day mechanically.

In the singing-dancing-painting-gardening experiences just mentioned, we are not attuning consciously to prana, and yet we are spontaneously experiencing a harmony of all parts of our being. The ideal is to bring about that harmony consciously and constantly. The following article by Yogi Desai explains how to do that by practicing different kinds of awareness throughout the day.

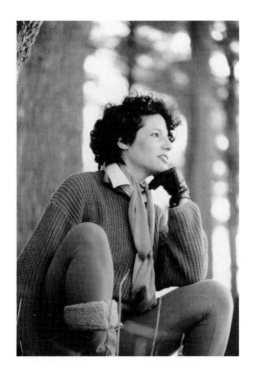
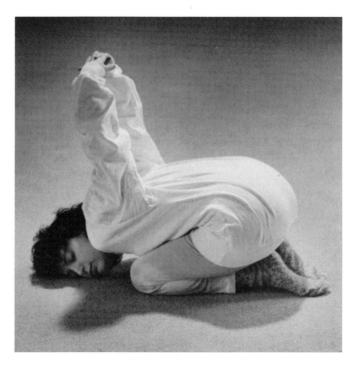
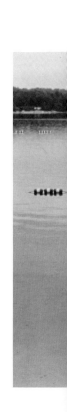

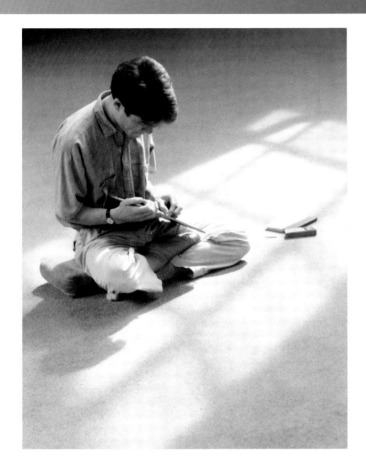

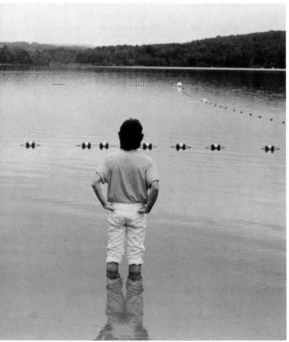

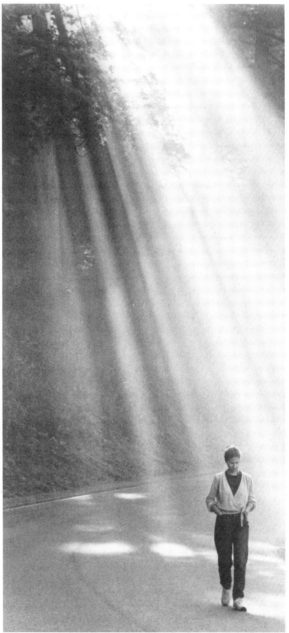

# THE MEDITATION OF LIVING PRANA
## by Yogi Amrit Desai

The purpose of applying the techniques of Kripalu Yoga to everyday life is to become more and more sensitive and attuned to your prana. Then every movement and thought becomes harmonious and relaxed, and your whole life becomes a meditation. It is called "the meditation of living prana."

How can you do that? By applying each individual stage of Kripalu Yoga to your daily life and bringing the same awareness and concentration to your everyday movements as you do to a yoga posture.

We perform yoga postures with awareness and attention because they are different from the way we move in everyday life; they are special, unusual. Most of us perform our normal daily activities, however, in a mechanical way. We have no awareness of what we are doing or how we are doing it, because the actions required are familiar and habitual.

Kripalu Yoga helps you break that mechanicalness and become fully conscious and aware of each action. Then you can choose to perform the actions that are necessary, in a way that is harmonious with your prana, thus multiplying the energy you have at your disposal and remaining deeply relaxed no matter what you are doing. That is the meditation of living prana and it is the highest, most holistic way of life.

## Stage 1 — Recognizing and Using the Postures of Daily Life

### FIRST: BECOME AWARE OF YOUR POSTURE AND RELAX

The first stage of Kripalu Yoga is perfecting the postures, but formal postures are only one medium of expression for Kripalu Yoga. If you raise your hands in a certain way it can be an expression of Kripalu Yoga also. So the first way to use your knowledge of Kripalu Yoga in your daily life is to become aware of the many different "postures" you assume throughout the day.

Freeze where you are right now. You are in a posture. You will change that posture often throughout the day to fit the needs of your body. The changes will be automatically regulated by your prana (if you don't block it by lack of attunement) rather than by your conscious mind.

As much as possible during the day, become aware of how prana, as expressed in the sensations in your body, wants to regulate your posture. Follow its guidance. Move, sit, or stand in the way that feels good to your body, whenever practical.

Of course there are places where you cannot assume the posture that feels best to you. For example, your prana may tell you to lie down, but if you are in your office you probably can't do that! At such times, simply maintain whatever posture is appropriate, but do it with relaxed awareness. Then, even if you cannot follow your prana, you are at least more aware of its needs.

If you can remain aware of your posture, you will be very relaxed and prana will flow freely through your body. Awareness of your body position and conscious relaxation of your body throughout the day, as often as you remember it, is practicing Kripalu Yoga, Stage One, all day long.

Whenever you become fully conscious of your body position, you will immediately experience relaxation and a flow of energy because you are listening to your prana much more closely than before. You will become extremely aware of your presence, your form, and your communication with your body and your surroundings.

This is how Kripalu Yoga can help to increase your awareness all day long. Do whatever you are doing with awareness, in a very relaxed way, and notice how much tension you drop when you consciously relax your movements. In other words, be conscious as often as you can while you are doing different things during the day.

For example, be aware of how the natural flow of energy is carrying you when you walk, and you will see the difference. Or, if you are changing your clothes, become aware of every position you assume. You'll be amazed at what happens to you. You'll be changing postures, and those postures will be unique when you do them with consciousness.

We all move our bodies through many different positions all day long, but hardly ever with conscious awareness. Kripalu Yoga is a method of interjecting awareness into every mechanical action that you are performing. That is very powerful.

### SECOND: CHANGE YOUR POSTURE TO CHANGE YOUR MOOD

The second way to use postures in everyday life is to change your posture consciously whenever you become aware that it is expressing an emotion or attitude that is not one you want to foster. Each posture expresses a certain feeling, and correcting it will change how you feel.

For example, if you are feeling depressed or frustrated, become aware of how you are walking. You walk in a different way. Your back begins to slump, you head droops a little so that you are looking down at the ground rather than straight ahead. At such times, use your awareness to pull up your physical center of gravity, which your emotions are pulling down. Consciously straighten your body and walk tall. Again you are using Kripalu Yoga, because Kripalu Yoga is one way of not allowing your emotions to take over your mind. Instead, constantly attune your mind to your prana, which is your Higher Self, and use conscious awareness to lift yourself out of negative feelings by changing your posture. When you are feeling depressed, anxious, frustrated, or any other negative emotion, just adjust your posture and walk straight, in a relaxed way, and see what happens.

Dress, too, has an important influence on how you feel. Never allow yourself to dress in an ugly or shabby way, especially when you're not feeling good. Instead, take a bath or shower, put on clean clothes, and then walk out with your head held high. Even put on an artificial smile if you have to. You are not being dishonest, because you are doing it consciously for a specific, good purpose.

In other words, if you haven't enough control yet over your inner mechanisms to feel good, use the support of every external means in your power. As you create a positive vibration all around you, other people will begin to feed you positive energy in return, and that will also help to change your energy.

There is nothing phoney about this, because you are doing it consciously. You are not doing it mechanically or for any false motivation. You are not trying to hide anything. You are simply making conscious use of every means at your disposal to come out of a negative experience.

### THIRD:
### LET YOUR THOUGHTS FOLLOW YOUR POSTURE

There is a third way you can use the postures and positions of your body to heighten your consciousness. An example describes it best: When you are reclining, consciously recline and feel deeply rested. Don't think about something else that involves sitting up and walking.

Have you seen a cat when it is resting? It just lies there, totally relaxed, and yet, when it wants to jump, it moves like lightening. So be like a cat: when you are sitting, sit with your mind too. When you are walking, walk. When you are lying, lie down. When you are working, work.

In other words, your posture will help you to get in touch with wherever you are and to stay grounded in it, to fully accept it. It will help you bring your mind and body into harmony.

Have you noticed people who, when they are sitting and talking to you, always look as if they are ready to leap to their feet? They spend almost as much energy as if they were actually running, and that is a waste.

Often when people are sitting, they are thinking of doing something else, so there is a split between the mind and body. The thoughts in the mind are at variance with the posture, causing the body to lose energy.

If you use your postures for awareness, by bringing your thoughts into harmony with your body position, you will be able to cut off that unnecessary wastage of energy. As a result, you will be relaxed and your energy will always be high. You'll be able to do effectively whatever you want to do.

### IN SUMMARY:
### USE POSTURE TO ATTUNE TO PRANA

So use your work with yoga postures as an model of how to consciously attune your thoughts to your body. It will enable you to be more relaxed and yet alert, living more naturally and in accord with the higher energy of prana rather than the false, restless energy of the individual mind and ego.

Many people are impressed by the achievements of those who are prominent in their fields. Often, I am not impressed. I see that most of the time those people draw their energy from ego. All their accomplishments are for the rest of the world and perhaps for history, but do not fulfill their inner selves.

What good is it when you have external accomplishments and everyone saying how wonderful you are, but you don't feel wonderful? Instead you feel unsatisfied, unfulfilled, or unhealthy.

Kripalu Yoga teaches you how to become more fulfilled by attuning to prana and becoming free of the grip of the ego. Awareness of body postures is an important beginning.

## Stage 2 — Using the Breath

The second way to use Kripalu Yoga to attune to prana is to become aware of your breathing during the day. Become aware of how you are breathing right now. Feel your breath flowing in and out. You are again making contact with your prana, this time through breath. You are once more becoming fully aware of your body in relation to the surrounding elements.

Life comes to us as physical experience rather than as thoughts, so the body is the only medium we have to experience life. As soon as we attend to our breath and regulate it, extraneous thoughts fade out, leaving the mind centered and able to take in what we are experiencing in the moment.

Whenever you are emotional, your breathing becomes shallow and irregular. As soon as you become aware of it, you will automatically want to breathe more deeply, regularly, and slowly, because that is the natural way of breathing. It is how children and animals breathe when they are resting.

When you breathe slowly and deeply, you are taking in more prana from the air and balancing your mind and emotions. Almost instantly, you will feel a calmness, and after you have practiced conscious breathing for a while, you will begin to experience a sense of mastery over your emotions. You will know that no outside force needs to affect you — that your reactions are all within your control.

You will accumulate tremendous amounts of energy by breath awareness. Not only do you breathe in more energy, you also dissipate less energy by getting less emotional. So breath awareness, as taught in Kripalu Yoga, is another way of establishing yourself in prana consciousness.

## Stage 3 — Slowing Down and Letting Your Mind Match the Speed of Your Movement

In the third stage of Kripalu Yoga, the body postures are done in extremely slow motion. To practice that stage in daily life, simply slow down everything you do. Give yourself time. If you are putting on your shirt, do it in slow motion. When you are putting on your shoes, do so very slowly and consciously.

Allow your actions to come from your conscious awareness, rather than from mechanical habits. This awareness will help you change your habits. Even if you just seem to be going from one habit to another, that's fine. The next one is at least a new habit and, in the meantime, you have learned a new awareness: how to change old habits.

Human beings are creatures of habit. Until we are enlightened, we will have habits. But awareness grows, and the technique of slowing everything down is helpful. For example, every time you get into your car, there is a specific, habitual way you do it. Consciously change that the next time you get in.

The whole point of slowing down is to perform every movement gracefully and flowingly without a jerk or suddenness. That slowness and flowingness of movement conserves energy and brings another kind of awareness to everything you do. Slow down even more, or actually stop before you begin a new activity.

If you drive a car, for example, and are in the habit of driving at seventy miles an hour, stop and ask yourself if you really want or need to drive that fast. Become aware of the tension created in your body by the need for increased alertness at that speed and by the fear of being caught.

Time your journey to see how much time you actually save by going seventy miles an hour, as opposed to fifty-five. If you save seven minutes, ask yourself the question "Is all the tension worth it, to save seven

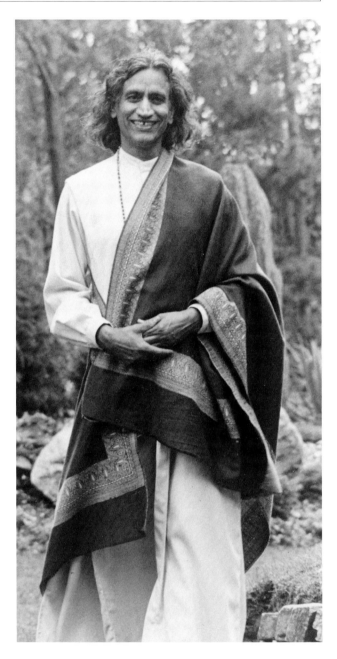

minutes?" If your answer is "no," consciously alter your habitual behavior and slow down your driving.

The second technique to foster awareness at Stage Three is to think slowly when you are moving slowly. In other words, be with your speed. When you are driving at fifty-five miles an hour, consciously accept that speed and don't wish you were going seventy, because then you will experience a fifteen-mile-an-hour tension.

Use your slowness to become conscious of your habits and to change them. Whether you are talking or walking, consciously slow down. Slow down your speech and listen to it. Slow down your walking and feel every movement.

As soon as you slow down, your prana will take over. You will move from consciousness, rather than from the mechanical part of your mind. And you'll begin to feel very relaxed, because when you slow down, you automatically drop into a relaxed state and into your feeling center.

All that happens spontaneously: you don't have to know how to do it. Your consciousness comes alive at once. Your awareness comes alive. Slowing down is a powerful way to train your awareness.

## Stage 4 — Affirming Life

The fourth stage of Kripalu Yoga is holding the posture and using creative visualization with it. To make use of that technique in your daily life, begin to observe everything you do and affirm it with a conscious statement.

For example, right now, as you read, consciously affirm and acknowledge to yourself "I am enjoying these teachings thoroughly; they are speaking directly to my heart and transforming my life. They are going into me very deeply."

Using affirmations in your life means being consciously aware, at every moment, of the good things that are happening to you and acknowledging them. So often we let the good things slip by us, taking them for granted, yet when unpleasant things are happening we become very conscious of them and complain loudly.

So affirm the good things that are already happening to you. This is what makes Kripalu affirmations very different from suggestion or self-hypnosis, in which you try to convince yourself of something that is not actually happening: Kripalu affirmations are statements of truth. And this technique, like the others, can be applied all day long.

Let's say that you are in a traffic jam, for example, and can't go as fast as you'd like. Just sit back, relax your posture, and acknowledge "There is nothing I can do at this time about the speed I am traveling, so here I am and that's fine. I'll take advantage of the situation by using the time to relax." That's your affirmation: simply acknowledging and accepting exactly what is happening, without frustration.

Prana affirmations are those made within the scope of existing conditions and situations. In following prana you are not trying to change the existing situation, you are learning to flow with it. You are simply affirming it, by being consciously aware of the good side of what is happening, and verbally acknowledging it, either mentally or aloud.

It is such a simple technique, yet it can change your life. You will have so much energy at the end of the day. Often you are tired because you have spent so much energy in mentally fighting things that cannot be changed, in not accepting what is.

## Stage 5 — Flowing with Life
### THE HEART OF THE KRIPALU APPROACH

Finally, the fifth stage of Kripalu Yoga is the posture flow. And if you practice, throughout the day, all the awarenesses outlined here, you will begin to experience yourself flowing through life.

Whether things happen the way you want or not, you will just flow through it, accepting everything that comes. You will not resist anything, mentally or emotionally. You will not fight anything. You will always work with it, not against it.

Your mind will become very clear. You will just have to ask yourself "What is the next thing that I need to do?" And you will be able to do it effortlessly. You will never be clogged with thoughts from previous moments; you will be fresh because your mind is in harmony with your prana.

You will do what you need to do, not what fulfills the dreams of your ego. You will sleep when you are sleepy and eat when you are hungry; you will rest when you are tired. You will follow whatever messages come naturally from prana. You will flow with life, always content, always relaxed. That is the Kripalu Approach to life. That is the meditation of living prana.

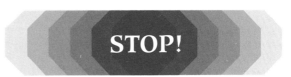

STOP!

How aware are you of your body messages right now? How are you feeling? Is there tension, stiffness, or tiredness in any part of your body? Do you need to get up and stretch? Take some deep breaths? Relax your shoulders? Rest your eyes? Rest your mind? Close your eyes for a minute and take some long, slow, deep breaths to enable you to get in touch with your experience. Then respond to what your body is asking you to do.

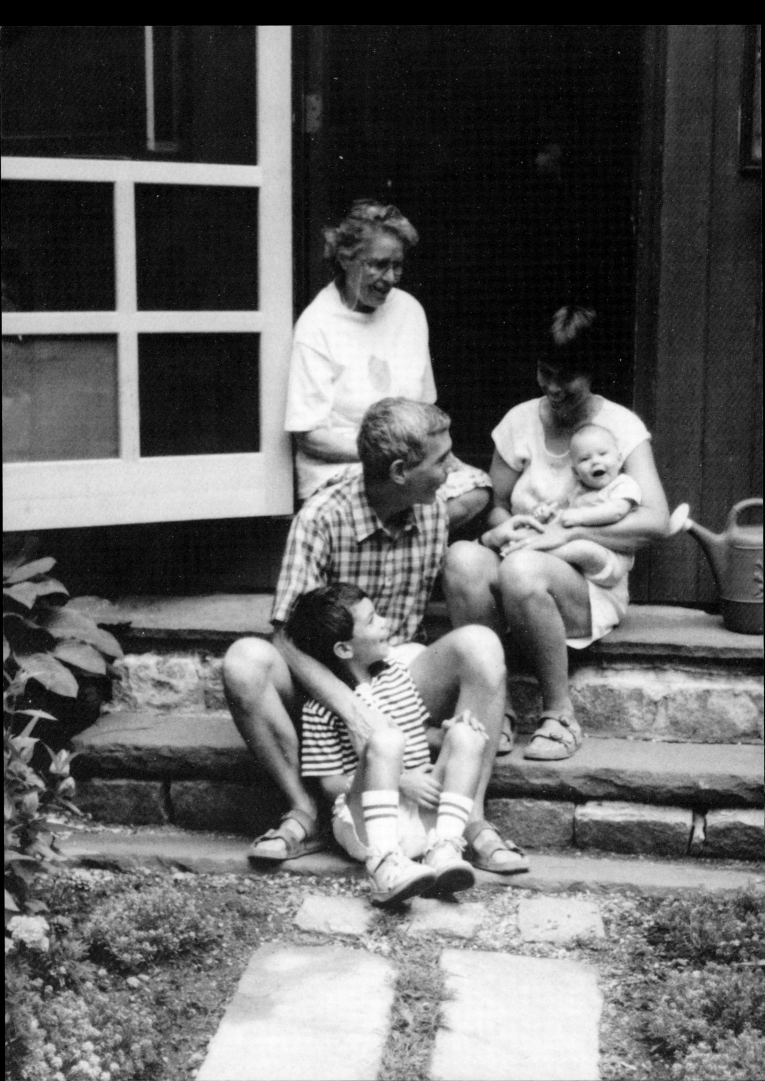

# The Eighth Pathway

creating a supportive lifestyle

# Holistic Health Involves Your Whole Life

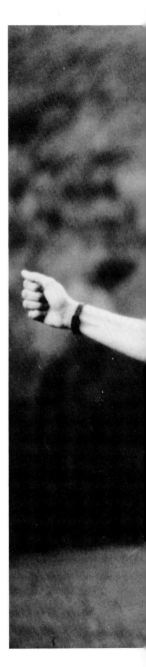

We have now come full circle to the point where we started this book: holistic health is the sum of how you live your whole life. The premise of the Kripalu Approach to health is, in the words of Yogi Desai: "You can't change your life without involving your life in the change."

This final chapter, then, explores the questions "How well does my present lifestyle support my aspiration for health and wholeness of body, mind, and spirit?" and "How can I modify my lifestyle so that it becomes even more supportive of my aspirations?"

There are three major elements involved in creating a supportive lifestyle, so the chapter is broken into three sections:

A. Your actions

B. Your environment

C. Your relationships

In reality those elements are not separate but interdependent. For instance, the people you relate to are both a consequence of and a part of your environment. So each area functions as a distinct element of support that can be focused on independently to bring about change, and yet that change will not be optimally effective unless the other areas are brought into alignment.

For example, you may seem to be doing all the right things for your life that are within your power, but if your environment is inconsistent with your needs and aspirations, your progress will be limited. Conversely, you may be in a totally supportive environment, but if your actions are not geared toward nurturing your health, you will not benefit much. And if your relationships are not harmonious and appropriate, your growth in other areas may be slower.

The Eighth Pathway addresses all the activities, relationships, and environment that influence your health and well-being, and how those factors can be modified in specific ways to bring your lifestyle into better alignment with your health goals.

So we will talk about changes you may choose to make, now or at a time in the future. Remember, there are no "shoulds" in the Kripalu Approach. As Yogi Desai has said: "A life of holistic health is not a life of giving up what you think you want; it is a life lived in the fullness of knowing and having what you really want."

Let's begin with the area in which you have the greatest immediate control: your personal actions and activities.

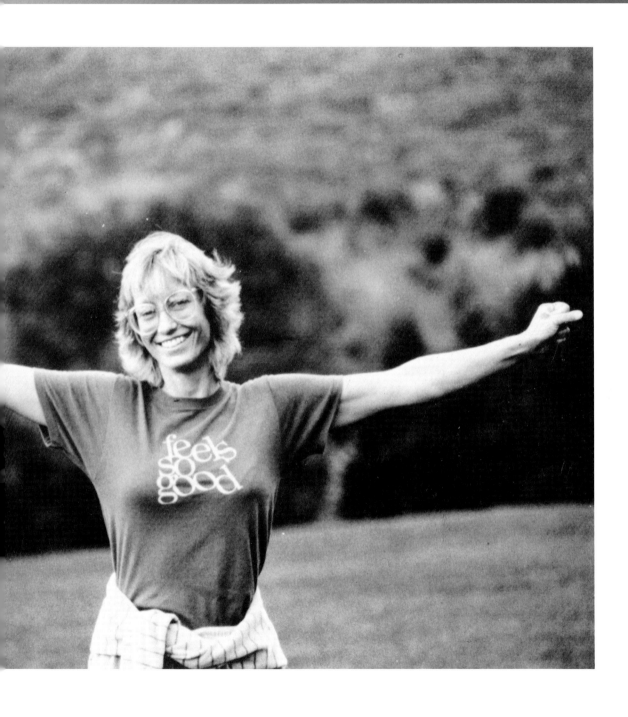

# Your Actions

First, review each of the Self-Discovery Experiences you have completed, with particular attention to the first one, "Check Your Holistic Health Quotient." See what you have learned from each one in terms of how well your actions and activities contribute to your experience of health and harmonious body-mind-spirit integration.

Notice how you feel about each area of activity: How interested are you in working on it? How much does it appeal to you? Do you feel you would enjoy it and find it fun? Or do you feel that you are not ready for it yet? Pay particular attention to the "Adjustment" sections, where you have outlined possible ways in which you might want to change your current behavior.

Now you are ready for action! Probably you have already been implementing some of these techniques into your daily life. The next step is to develop an integrated, balanced plan of action, so that you do not take on too much and become discouraged, or concentrate too much in one area and create new imbalances to replace the old ones.

The first and most important step is to set priorities: to establish what is most important to you and the order in which you want to proceed. The following chart should help with that.

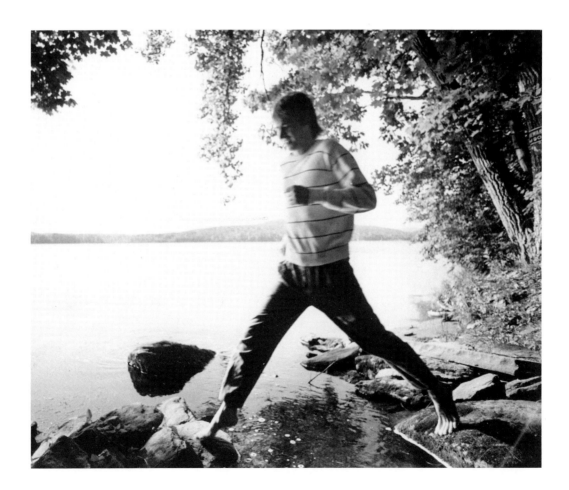

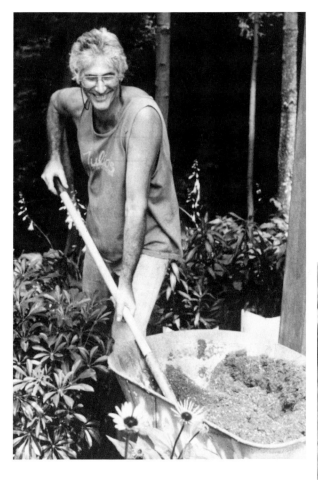

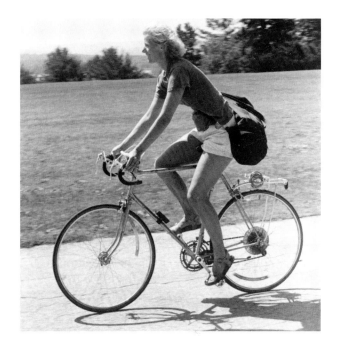

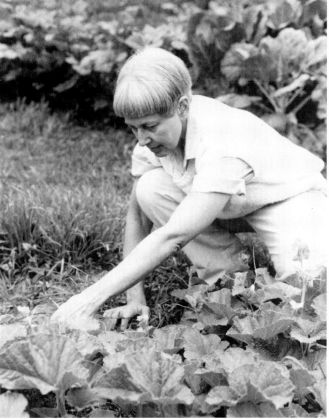

# Setting Priorities

Review the following list of possible growth objectives and place a mark in the box that indicates the priority of that objective for you. Try not to evaluate the objectives in terms of what you think you should do, but in terms of what you want to do and would feel good to you to work on.

| | Top priority | Very important | Important but can wait | Not right now |
|---|---|---|---|---|
| 1. Improving my diet | | | | |
| 2. Getting more exercise | | | | |
| 3. Taking up yoga (or increasing the length and/or frequency of my yoga sessions) | | | | |
| 4. Adjusting my sleep/rest habits for greater regularity | | | | |
| 5. Beginning the use of conscious relaxation techniques (or increasing the length and/or frequency of my conscious relaxations) | | | | |
| 6. Establishing group support for health practices and spiritual activity | | | | |
| 7. Practicing self-observation regularly through journal, introspection, and/or other means | | | | |
| 8. Beginning the regular use of a cleansing diet, fasting, and/or other types of purification (or increasing the length and/or frequency of same) | | | | |
| 9. Beginning to meditate (or increasing the length and/or frequency of my meditations) | | | | |
| 10. Cultivating more relaxed, harmonious relationships and attitudes at work | | | | |
| 11. Allowing the child in me more room for creativity and play | | | | |
| 12. Improving my communications and relationships with friends and family | | | | |
| 13. Achieving greater inner attunement | | | | |
| 14. Other: | | | | |
| 15. Other: | | | | |

1. Now that you have set your priorities, review your list of Top Priority growth items and pick one that you especially want to focus on in the immediate future. If you did not have any top priority items then choose from the Very Important items.

   In choosing your growth goal, don't pick something that you know would be very difficult to change. For example, you may want to eat moderately, but you may also know that it is too much to expect of yourself right now, given everything that is going on in your life. Choose something that you feel you could change with a moderate amount of effort and concentration. For example, you may decide that scheduling a conscious relaxation on a daily basis is a growth goal that is within your capacity to accomplish right now. Once having mastered relaxation, you will be in a better position to make a change in your eating habits.

2. After choosing your priority, make a very specific list of all of the possible ways you could go about acquiring the new habit. In the case of practicing daily relaxation, you might have some of the following as part of your list.

   I could practice
   - before lunch for fifteen minutes.
   - before dinner for fifteen minutes.
   - in the bus to and from work.
   - as I wait for meetings to begin.
   - as I stand in line at the lunch counter.

3. Go over your list and pick the one approach that is most practical and realistic for you to have some degree of success with, given your current life conditions. You may decide to practice relaxation everyday before lunch, because you know that relaxing before dinner is impossible with your children and the dog around.

4. Choose a length of time (one or two weeks) to practice the new behavior, with the goal of reviewing how you are doing at the end of that time. It helps to keep a daily journal of your experiences in acquiring your new skill.

   A sample entry might read "Tried relaxation for twelve minutes today in office but was interrupted by secretary. Will have to put 'do not disturb' note on my door tomorrow." As you make entries, you learn how you are doing and your journal becomes a record of your accomplishments and joys in growth.

5. Most important of all, as you embark on your journey learn to cultivate an attitude of acceptance of yourself and whatever happens. Whenever we try something new, we meet our inner resistance. There is a part of every one of us that wants to grow and change and be a better person.

   There is also a hidden part of us that, deep down, doesn't want to change, but prefers the ease and security of our present known habits and way of life. That part fears the unknown — or is simply lazy! We can only overcome our resistance by first accepting it (which means accepting ourselves) and learning to work with and through it.

   Everything that happens to us can enhance our awareness and, consequently, our joy of living — if we accept it. Remember the THREE A's formula for achieving well-being: If I'm AWARE of who I am, and I ACCEPT the self I see, then I have all I'll ever need to ADJUST my behavior and reveal the REAL ME.

   Whatever happens, remain inspired. In order to make lasting changes in the direction of more beneficial health habits, you will need to re-inspire yourself again and again to be constant in your commitment and your efforts and full of enthusiasm for the journey you are undertaking.

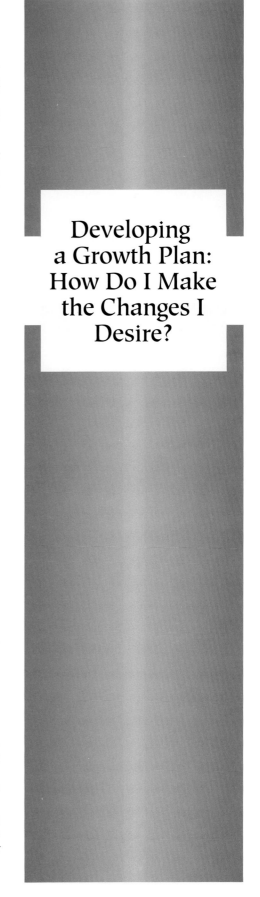

# Developing a Growth Plan: How Do I Make the Changes I Desire?

# Your Environment

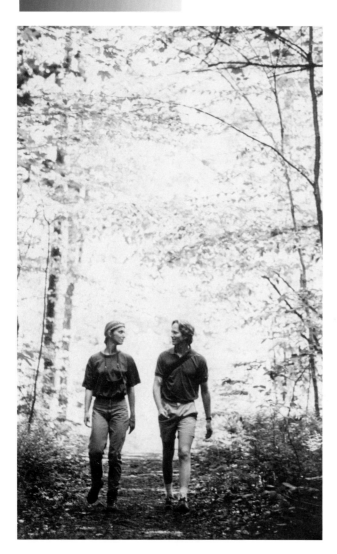

## The Surroundings

Now that you have decided on a specific plan of action for your daily activities, let's take a look at your environment, or more accurately, your environments, for you pass through many different environments everyday.

The dictionary defines *environment* as "the external conditions in which a person or organism lives." It's obvious that you are a person living in an environment, but have you thought of yourself an an "organism"? That implies something vital, sensitive, and easily affected by external conditions. An organism takes in and is nourished by the things that surround it.

Remember learning in biology about the life of a simple cell and how it takes in nutrients through a process of absorption called osmosis? Reflect on the fact that your body is nothing more or less than a vast conglomeration of millions of cells that are constantly absorbing nutrients of all kinds from their environment, and you will understand better just how sensitive your body is.

How does that absorption happen? Principally it happens through the medium of our five senses: not only are we hearing, seeing, tasting, and smelling the world around us, we are also feeling it with every inch of our skin.

## Our Surroundings Are Spiritual Food

Another important characteristic of a living organism is that it constantly adapts to its environment. That is how the whole process of evolution occurs. In the same way, the human body is constantly being called upon to adjust and adapt to its surroundings.

It is important for our health that our physiological adaptations be in the right direction; that is, that the adaptation required be one favorable to health. The same is true for psychological impressions created by external stimuli: just as we need to be careful of what food we eat to nourish our bodies, so we need to be aware and careful of what impressions we allow ourselves to take in to nourish our minds and emotions.

Since our senses tend not to discriminate, but to take in all that surrounds them, whether or not we are aware of it, it follows that we must be very discriminating in terms of the environments into which we place ourselves.

We have to decide what is supportive, in terms of environment, and what is not. Returning to the dictionary, we find that *supportive* means "that which holds or props up; provides for the needs of; helps, approves of; encourages." So a supportive environment is one that provides for the needs of the organism — your body, mind, and spirit — and encourages your total growth.

## Nourish Yourself with Healthful Surroundings

For a moment picture yourself standing on a busy downtown street of a big city. Cars rush by, horns honk, exhaust fumes fill the air, people walk briskly past, litter lines the sidewalk, buildings tower above you, a myriad of neon signs invite you to buy this and

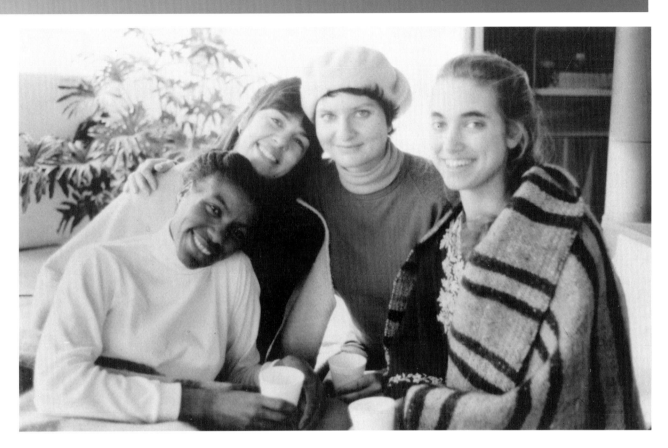

try that, and the smell of hot pretzels from a nearby vendor drifts past your nose.

All those impressions bombarding your senses are asking for an adjustment from the body; they demand adaptation or movement, action or reaction. That means that they are each placing energy demands on the body. No wonder the city dweller is often tired when he or she gets home.

Now visualize yourself in the country, walking along a tree-lined lane amidst quiet fields. All you hear are birds twittering, the occasional bark of a dog, and perhaps a distant chain-saw as the only sound of civilization. You're breathing fresh, cool air and a gentle breeze caresses your skin.

These examples are not given to condemn city life and encourage everyone to move to the country, but rather to illustrate a subtle point and to stimulate your awareness so that you can balance out the environments in which you spend your time.

The more external stimuli, the greater the energy demand on the body. The more unhealthy the surroundings, the more the body is called on to adapt.

In the first visualization, chances are you felt yourself tensing slightly to combat the noise and fumes. In the second, you probably felt yourself relaxing.

Relaxation is free-flowing energy and tension is blockage and waste of energy. Environment is absolutely key to the Kripalu Approach, which teaches that conserving prana energy and being relaxed will lead to holistic health. A truly supportive environment feeds our senses with its harmony, order, and peace.

Such an environment could be a quiet country setting, but it could also be a homey kitchen redolent with the smell of lovingly prepared food. It could be a tidy desk with an inspiring picture; a meditation room simply furnished in harmonious, quiet colors; or a brisk walk to work through the relative quiet of pre-rush hour streets.

Those are just a few examples of supportive environments in which we could feel peaceful and relaxed and in tune with our inner needs.

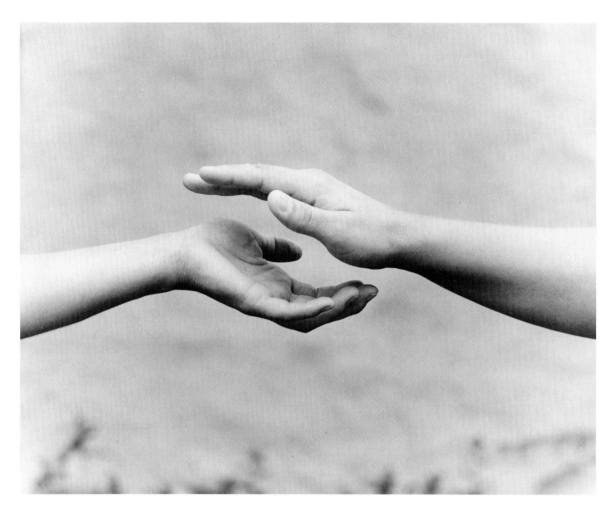

## The Social Aspect of Environment

A supportive environment could also be a circle of friends sharing their happiness and sorrow together, because it is not only our physical environment that affects us, it is also the people with whom we interact in that environment. That means we must consider the people we spend time with (and how we spend that time) in terms of how those interactions contribute to our growth.

This is not a way to advocate selfishness — at least, not in the usual sense of the word (see the following section on Relationships). It is rather an invitation to evaluate seriously whether certain social situations are really supportive of our health ideals and, if not, what to do about them.

Let's say you have decided that one of your priorities is to eat a more natural, wholesome, healthy diet that is free of refined or processed foods containing chemical additives. If you usually find yourself eating meals with a group of people who have different needs and awarenesses and prefer what you regard as

unhealthy, nutritionless food, you will experience conflicting desires and a resultant energy loss.

You may want to be with those people, or at least not to lose their friendship, yet you don't feel good when you eat what you have decided is not good for your body. The same thing will happen if you prefer not to drink alcohol, yet you spend a lot of time with people who like to go to bars; or if you've given up smoking and yet many situations involve your being in smoke-filled environments.

Of course, you may not always seem to have choice. If you work in an office where everyone smokes, it might seem to be a no-choice situation. On the other hand, you can always ask yourself "Do I have a choice? Could I work somewhere else? What is most important to me?"

With the idea of choice in mind, complete the Self-Discovery Experience that follows to see if it reveals to you some new choices you might make in order to create for yourself a more supportive environment.

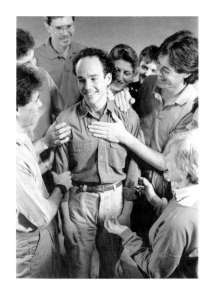
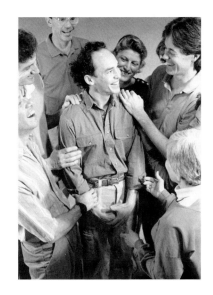
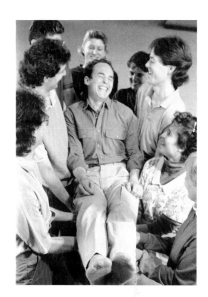
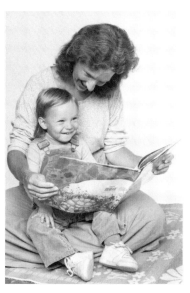
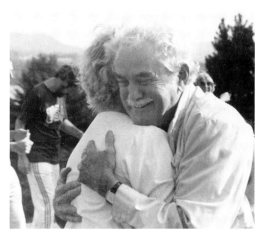
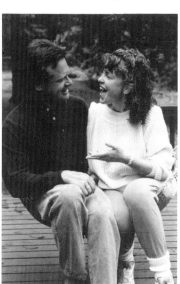
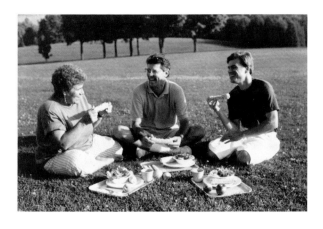
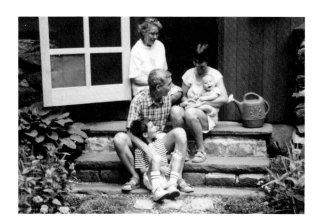

## Self-Discovery Experience

## 15

### How well does your environment support your health?

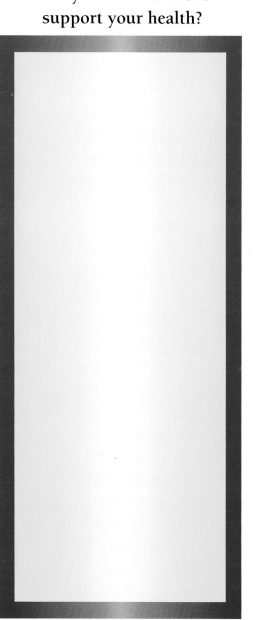

### Awareness

1. Sit quietly for a moment with your eyes closed and review all the different environments in which you find yourself in the course of a typical day. Open your eyes and list them on a sheet of paper, starting with the environment of your bedroom when you wake in the morning and passing through your house, your car or perhaps a subway, your work environment, and whatever else, until you return to your bed at night.

2. Circle the environments you like best and which you feel best support your growth.

3. Look over the circled items. Close your eyes and place yourself in each one for a few minutes. Really experience it. See and feel the people and the setting, hear the voices, taste the tastes, smell the odors.

4. After each visualization, list the feelings that came up in you.

5. Reflect for a moment on the characteristics that your favorite environments have in common. In what ways are they similar? Write down the qualities that come to you.

6. Think about the people in those environments, then list them, describing how you feel about each one, the quality of the time you spend together, and the level of communication between you.

7. Circle the names of the people you most enjoy being with and who, in your opinion, support your health and growth.

## Acceptance

8. Take a look at the environments and names you didn't circle. Ask yourself for each one: "Do I wish to avoid this environment, person, or situation? If so, do I have a choice: can I avoid it/him or her? If I can, why don't I? What do I stand to lose? What do I get that I feel I need from that environment, person, or situation? How else can I meet that need?"

9. Select one of the environments where you experience conflicting needs and feelings. Enter into it, with your eyes closed, through creative visualization and explore your feelings and perceived needs. Ask yourself: "What do I really want in my life? How can I achieve that through this situation? What in this situation seems to be pulling me away from my main purpose? Why do I allow that?"

10. For other situations that do not seem supportive of your holistic health and spiritual growth, ask yourself: "What other needs am I trying to meet? Are those needs really important to me?" If they do feel important to you at this time, ask "How else can I meet them?"

   In the process of that kind of questioning, you will probably see that in many such situations the underlying need is either for social interaction (fun, companionship, or friendship) or for relaxation.

   What you may also see is that, in some cases, the apparently natural human need for companionship is in reality a desire for external acceptance and approval or a superficial cure for the loneliness that comes from not truly being in touch with your inner self.

   The need for relaxation is genuine, too, and yet true, natural relaxation does not usually result from the kinds of situations and activities that we have come to associate with that term, such as social eating, drinking, and group activities.

11. Now ask yourself about each of your social relationships: "Is this relationship a meaningful friendship that helps both/all of us to grow and learn? Or is it relatively superficial, simply filling the need to be with another person or to kill time? Does it just exist because we do certain things together? If there weren't before-dinner drinks, cups of coffee, and gourmet meals, would we still want to spend time with each other?"

   These are hard questions to ask of ourselves, and yet, if we want our environment to support our growth in every possible way, it is necessary that we ask them.

## Adjustment

Now it is simply a question of recognizing and accepting your own inner priorities, the urgings of prana as they speak to you through your body and intuitive feelings. Once you have seen where the conflicts lie in your environment and social situations, you will be able to begin to make the necessary adjustments to your lifestyle.

12. List the specific changes that you can make easily.

13. Now write down some ways in which you can gradually make other, more difficult changes, while keeping in harmony with those around you.

14. Review the situations in which you cannot realistically make changes at present and resolve to accept them willingly and open-heartedly.

   In order to facilitate the above process, it is important to be very clear about the pros and cons of each situation and to weigh them carefully. It is helpful to make two lists.

   It may be possible to change some factors, and yet, all things considered, more desirable not to make those changes right now. Look carefully to see where happy compromises are the best solution and impatience would cause unnecessary difficulties.

   For example, as a mother, you might wish to have your family become vegetarian. However, if you perceive that that could create tremendous strain on family relationships, it might be better to continue to serve meat, but begin to make it less important. You might introduce occasional meat substitutes, excitingly prepared, or simply serve more fowl and seafood and de-emphasize red meat.

   Everything depends on the situation and the people. The important thing is to be aware of and weigh the possible results of each action.

# GIVING AND RECEIVING
## by Yogi Amrit Desai

In today's world of self-centered and deteriorating relationships, love has become a very confused and misunderstood concept. Usually what is known as love is no more than attachment. Attachment and love are diametrically opposed qualities. They cannot exist simultaneously; they are mutually exclusive.

Real love makes no demands; it is free of expectations. We love simply for the sake of loving, for the pure joy of loving in and of itself. Love emanates from the center of peace and contentment within us.

In attachment our experience of love depends upon an outside person or object. There is a desired result to be gained by loving; there is a goal in the relationship. Attachment, then, is a contract or exchange. "If you do this, I will love you. If you stop doing it, I will no longer love you."

Thus, attachment becomes an emotional addiction, a dependence upon receiving a desired goal. When the goal is not achieved, what we have called love disappears and pain results.

When two people are attracted to each other, they each discover desirable qualities in the other and feel that the needs of both can be met in their relationship. Any differences that exist between them seem unimportant because the power of emotion is so strong.

The play of emotional attraction may continue for a long time, particularly during the premarriage and early marriage stages. Yet once those powerful emotions begin to settle, the differences they had overlooked begin to be apparent.

If sexual attraction is the glue that holds the relationship together, the relationship will wane as the thrill of emotion wanes. Other areas of growth may be ignored in the temporary fervor of sexual union. And sex may unwittingly be used to hide disagreements that arise, with the phrase "Let's kiss and make up" closing the door to real communication.

When pain caused by disharmony within a relationship is swallowed, resentful anger, disappointment, and frustration may lodge deep within each partner. Such disharmony can occur within any close relationship, but since marriage is the closest of all relationships, communication in marriage is considerably more intense.

## Loving from Our Inner Center of Contentment

When we truly love we take joy in others and feel compassion for them, but we do not look to them as the means of satisfying our emotional needs and addictions. We are aware that happiness is something we draw from the core of our being and then share with others, not demand from others.

Our inner core then becomes the source of our fulfillment. We do not need others, in the sense of being totally dependent on them, for our happiness. When we discover and learn to relate from that inner center of happiness and contentment, all who come near us receive our freely given gift of love.

There is only one way to receive love and that is to give love. Only when we give freely are we truly able to receive, for in giving we receive inner joy, and that joy is what we really wanted anyway! Many people mete out very carefully the love they give and watch closely to see if it is returned with equal measure.

In truth, not only is there no way to measure love, but love given with a desire for return is not even love: it is a contract. So if we want to be loved, we must give love totally, with no thought of receiving anything in return. Then we will experience the state of love, of being in love, rather than the act of giving or receiving love.

Love requires continuous practice. The best place to begin practicing is with ourselves, because everything depends on our attitudes toward life. We need to change our habitual attitudes and ways of viewing the world in order to come to that center of inner fulfillment and joy.

As we progress in our mastery of love, we no longer reject anyone simply on the basis of our value systems or concepts of how they should be for us. We no longer entertain negative thoughts about others. Instead, we begin to live creatively, consciously developing in our relationships positive new attitudes, habits, and experiences.

When difficulties arise between us and someone else, the solution is to begin actively to recall and dwell on the beautiful qualities that we have recognized within the other person. As we continue to recall all that we have previously admired and loved in that person, we discover that our gestures, the words we speak, and the way we look at him or her begin to change.

Soon we will find that the other person instinctively begins to feel our acceptance and love without our ever expressing it in words. Confidence grows within the other that our outlook has become steady and positive, and that he or she is accepted and loved unconditionally. As the other person relaxes in the embrace of our new, non-demanding love, he or she also begins to change, and then any conflict can be easily resolved.

Words can never disguise a lack of love; that is why we need to change our thinking. If we constantly speak words of love to others and yet entertain negative thoughts, they will not be deceived. They need not be psychologists to read our hidden language. For that reason, it is essential to think only positive thoughts about anyone with whom we are having difficulty.

Such positive thinking is not a suppression of negativity; rather, it is a rechanneling process. Negative thoughts are recognized, acknowledged, and accepted as natural. Then we simply give them no more attention or energy.

As we develop a conscious pattern of honestly recognizing all that we admire within the other person, our positive thoughts will drown out negative ones just as light dispels the darkness in a room when you turn on the light switch. Positive thinking is the major secret of all good relations with others.

## Marriage as a Tool for Mutual Growth

A marriage relationship that has as its main purpose the physical, emotional, and spiritual growth of the partners enables a deep and lasting union to develop regardless of the outer changing circumstances.

As each partner learns to offer support in the most difficult times, as well as in the many times of joy and shared happiness, and works at entertaining only positive feelings about the partner, the growth that occurs far surpasses any outward support that could be received.

Honest and loving faith in each other establishes a chain reaction, for each opportunity in which one partner can give sincerely enables a warm and genuine exchange of gratitude. Feelings become totally supportive as each partner strives to be loving in all situations and avoids relying on the other to fulfill his or her emotional needs.

Paradoxically enough, all those needs will in reality be fulfilled, for the internal happiness and strength that comes from freely giving without expectations brings the experience of deep peace and contentment that was the original basic need anyway. The limited time that modern families are able to spend together will seem to become limitless between loving partners, for their

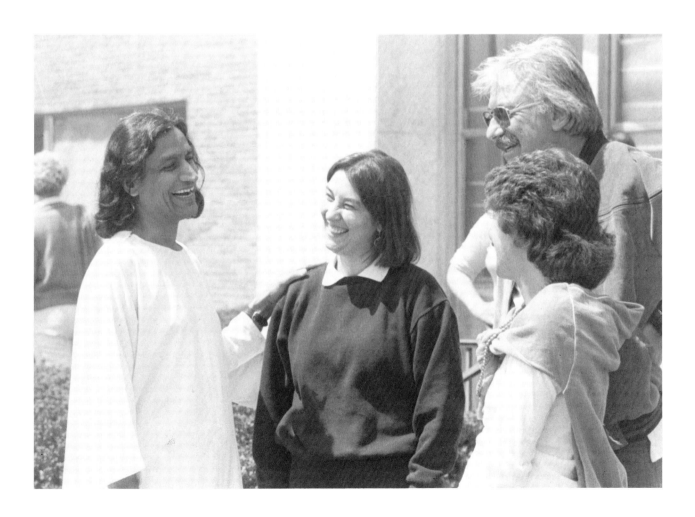

feeling of togetherness is an ongoing internal experience regardless of physical distance. Communication becomes loving, honest, and open; there is no need for fear as the relationship grows in the power of mutual giving.

## Giving Love is Giving Ourselves

When we give love, we are providing security to others. We are caring for them and providing them comfort and ease. As a result, we have no reason to experience tension or anxiety with others because we have made them so secure that they have no reason to do anything we might experience as threatening.

When we expect or demand something from others, we subconsciously set them up as a threat, because they are able to withhold whatever it is we seek from them. As a result, we fear not getting what we need from them and become defensive and self-protective.

Thus, providing loving security to others enables us to feel secure. Demanding security from others robs us of the security that is already present within us, just waiting to be uncovered. Anyone can create a false feeling of acceptance and belonging by demanding it from some outside source, but only a person of true depth and maturity can find acceptance within.

As you learn to accept yourself and to know that you are fine just as you are, with all your faults, you will naturally accept as they are your marriage partner and all others with whom you come in contact. Only then can you experience and give unconditional love that is free from fear, dependence, and attachment.

Your practice of unconditional love can start by accepting yourself and others at the same time. Eventually your love will begin to be reflected back to you as you grow in the experience of providing love to others without an expectation of return.

Remember that you can never love too much, but you can love too much in your own way, which may not be understood by the other. So when you love, you must do so in a way that can be understood and taken in by others. Then they won't feel threatened or imagine that you want something from them; they will recognize your love for what it is — a free gift.

## Simply Drop What Love Is Not

We don't need to know what unconditional love is in order to practice it; we simply need to know what love is not and then drop those non-love thoughts and actions from our lives. Deep in our hearts, we all know what is not loving. It is not loving to hate others, to be jealous of them, to compete with them, to want them to be different from the way they are.

We know that violence is not loving, so we usually do not perform acts of physical violence. Yet we do not often realize that we are constantly performing more subtle acts of violence through thoughts and actions that are nonaccepting of people (jealousy, competitiveness, the desire to change them).

When we are acting from love, we come up with creative solutions to difficult encounters by seeing objectively where we can change our experience of the external situation by changing something in ourselves. That constant adaptability and willingness to adjust is true unselfishness, which is the very essence of being loving.

We commit acts and thoughts of subtle violence on ourselves, too, every time we feel guilty or reject or blame ourselves. Catching those subtle thoughts and actions is a place to begin to practice love for ourselves. And it is only when we are able truly to love and accept ourselves as we are, unconditionally, that we will be able truly to love and accept others.

# In Conclusion

You have reached the end of this book and we hope that you now have a whole new and inspired set of tools to help you progress on your path to holistic health. You may feel as if you have made a new friend.

You have learned much about this new friend: his or her strengths and beauties, and endearing weaknesses and idiosyncrasies. We hope you have come to treasure and respect this new friend, in body, mind, and spirit. Certainly you will be continually amazed and delighted as you discover, probably daily, new things about him or her.

You have made this friend some promises, as you would in any relationship. You have promised always to listen to his or her needs, and to try your best to fulfill them. You have committed yourself to doing your utmost to help that friend maintain his or her health and to move together to higher levels of vibrant well-being.

You have promised to relax and play together, and to share your joys and sorrows. You have, above all, resolved never to forget or reject this friend, no matter what. For this friend is your very self.

We wish you wonder-filled adventures on your journey together.

We salute the light within you.

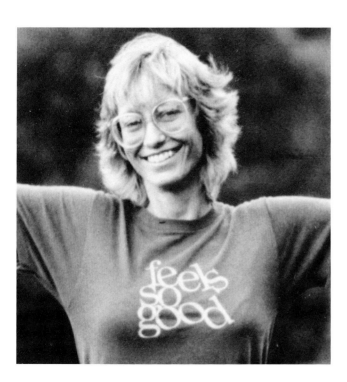

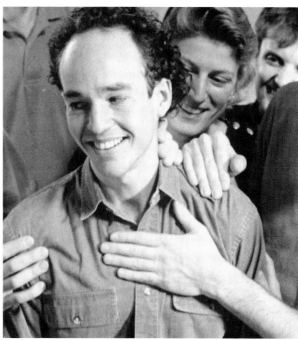

# Appendix

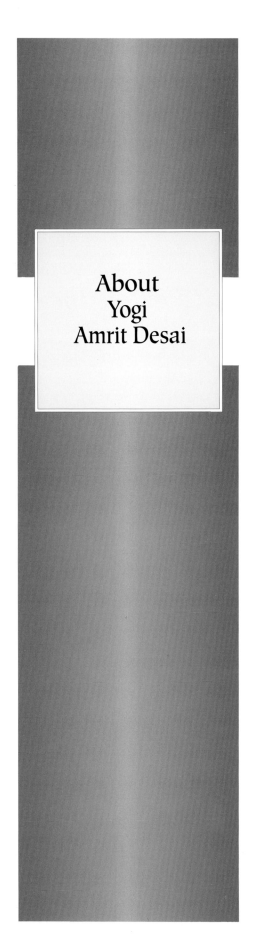

## About
## Yogi
## Amrit Desai

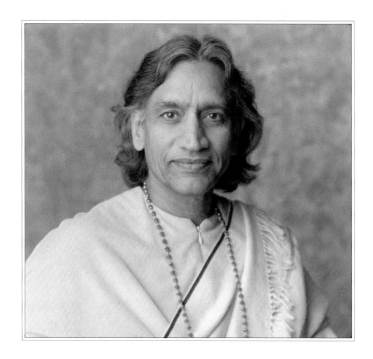

Yogi Amrit Desai is an internationally recognized authority on the yogic principles of self-transformation and holistic health. During his more than thirty years in the West, he has been honored repeatedly by the international yoga community with titles such as Doctor of Yogic Science and Jagadacharya (World Teacher).

One of Yogi Desai's outstanding contributions to humanity is his ongoing development of Kripalu Yoga, a unique yet authentic approach to the ancient science of yoga. Kripalu Yoga is a yoga of consciousness that focuses on integration of body, mind, and spirit. As a result, its principles can be applied to every aspect of life.

In developing Kripalu Yoga, Yogi Desai has drawn not only upon personal experience, but upon the profound teachings he received from his spiritual teacher, Swami Shri Kripalvanandji. It is for his revered teacher that Kripalu Yoga and Kripalu Center are named.

Kripalu Center was founded by Yogi Desai as a way of supporting people from all walks of life in their quest for greater health and personal growth. He inspires its staff of over two hundred fifty residents to model a lifestyle blending contemporary approaches to self-development with the traditional wisdom of yoga.

Yogi Desai travels much of the year, lecturing and answering questions on the art of holistic living. His very presence speaks powerfully of his approach, for he is the epitome of a healthy, joyful, self-actualized human being living at the peak of his potential.

When not traveling, Yogi Desai lives at Kripalu Center for Yoga and Health. For information on his seminar schedule, contact Seminars Department, Kripalu Center, Box 793, Lenox, MA 01240.

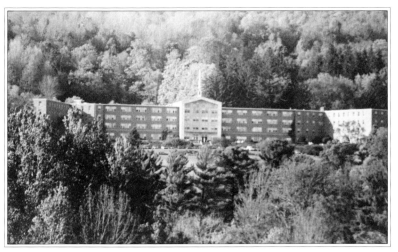

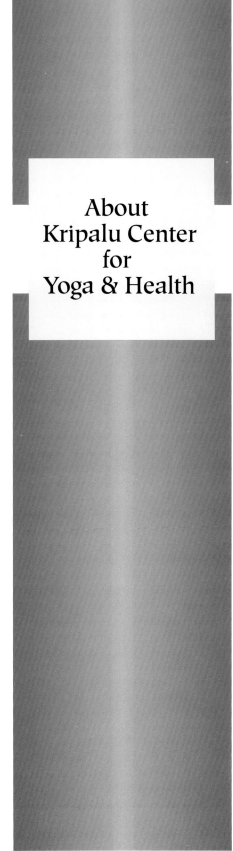

Kripalu Center is both a spiritual community and a world-renowned holistic educational facility. Located in the Berkshire hills of western Massachusetts, the Center is open year-round, offering programs and individual health services promoting the integration of body, mind, and spirit.

The basis of Kripalu's approach to health is the ancient and transformative science of yoga. Yogic principles maintain that physical health is not only a valuable asset in and of itself, but the foundation for emotional, mental, and spiritual development as well.

Programs at the Center combine the practice of authentic yogic disciplines with other, more contemporary approaches to personal growth. The combination provides not just intellectual understanding, but first-hand experiences that lead to radiant well-being and a greater sense of aliveness.

Kripalu offers programs in the areas of self-discovery, yoga, spiritual attunement, and bodywork. Guests may also choose a more unstructured schedule with as much variety and activity as desired.

Individual health services, available to Center guests and the general public, include sessions in Kripalu bodywork, energy balancing, Shiatsu, reflexology, and skin care. Kripalu also has two saunas and whirlpools for guest use. General facilities include a full range of comfortable accomodations, convenient lounges with stunning lake and mountain views, a book and gift shop, a natural foods kitchen and bakery, and spacious activity rooms for workshops and program sessions.

Kripalu Center is available to support you in the process you've begun with *Kripalu's Self Health Guide*. Programs, books, and tapes available through the Center can help deepen and extend your experience of renewed health and greater well-being. To receive our program calendar and guide, *The Kripalu Experience*, write Kripalu Center for Yoga and Health, Box 793, Lenox, MA 01240; or call 1-800-967-3577. For a helpful catalog of our products available by mail, call 1-800-967-7279.

Kripalu Center is a non-profit, federally tax-exempt organization.

# Index